# My other books:

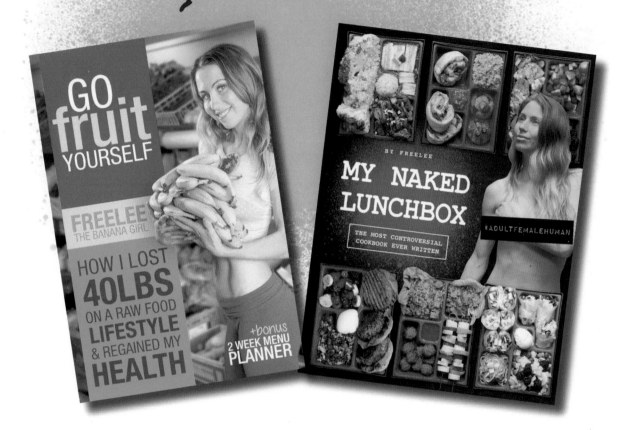

# thebananagirl.com

### DISCLAIMER

# TABLE OF CONTENTS

# RECIPES 153

# WELCOME FUTURE BANANA GIRL

Celebrate! You have just opened the book that is going to transform your body and mind forever.

It was no mistake you chose this book, it was obviously time. We both know you have been searching for a way out of the ugly, dieting world or to simply feel and look better. Subconsciously searching for a lifestyle that will allow you to eat as much as you want to and still look your best. A lifestyle that cares for your health as well as the health of the Planet and the animals too.

A lifestyle that just feels right. You know what I mean, Well THIS IS IT! This is the book that I wish I had picked up years ago when I was struggling with being overweight, sick and depressed , when I was so lost that suicide seemed like the best option. A life where purging was a daily event.

This book has been in creation my whole life, countless hours of trial and error have been channelled into it. I have lived through the starvation bikini plans, the Paleo death diets, the Hot Yoga, water fasting, you name it, I tried it. Now you can save a shitload of time, pain, cash and metabolic damage by simply reading this book and implementing the guidelines into your daily life. I have personally invested thousands of dollars into making this book what it is today and you can get it for the price of a night at the movies or a meal at a restaurant.

This is the ultimate investment in your future self. I look forward to hearing about your successes on RT4 and I am so happy to be able to introduce this book to you. I know you are ready to dive straight into this so lettuce begin. It's time to become the healthiest, happiest person you know! BOOM! Time to go fruit yourself. ;-)

Freelee

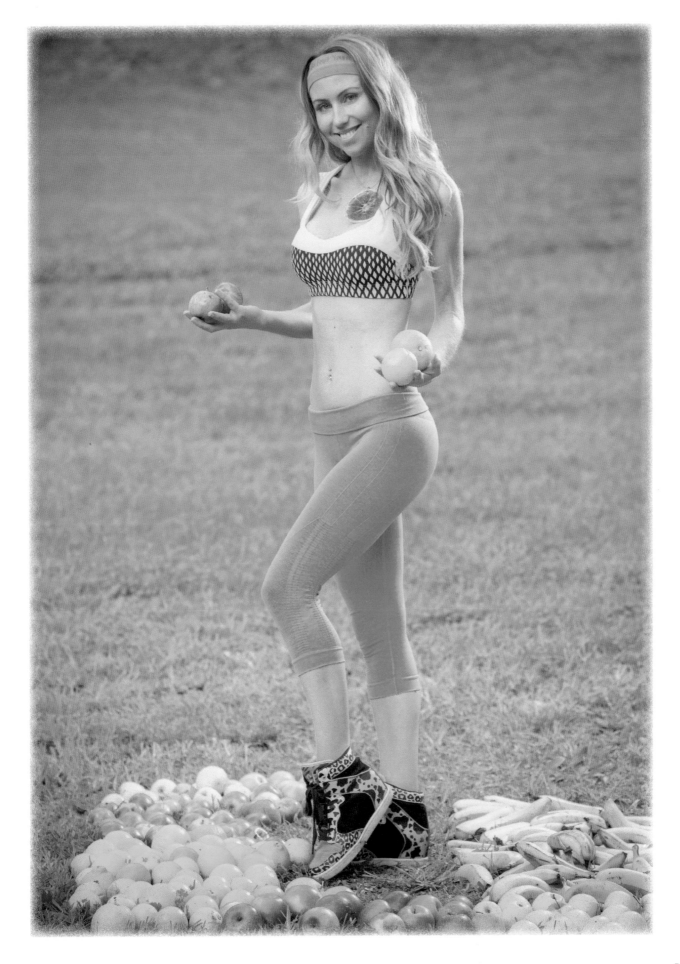

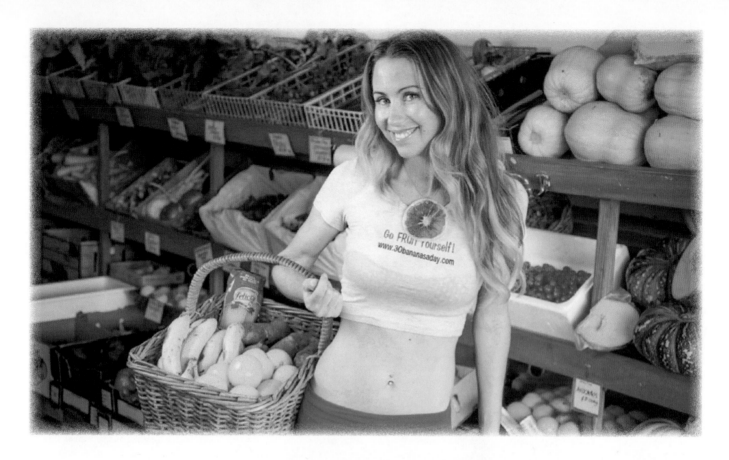

# JOIN THE BANANA GIRL COMMUNITY
# ON SOCIAL MEDIA

*First up, don't be a dummy and try to go this alone. Connect up with other banana girls doing the 30 day cleanse. Social media will always be the most convenient and efficient form of connecting with others, so I recommend you use the following hashtags and then check out who else is using them to say hey! :*

**#BGC30** - Banana Girl Cleanse 30 days
**#RAW24 -** 24 hrs of 100% raw food
**#RAWTILL4 -** Already with nearly a million tags
**#RT4**
**#BANANAGIRL**

Connecting with others will help you stay on track with your 30 day cleanse. Of course, the aim is for you to adopt the RT4 lifestyle - however a 30 day introduction is a great start. I recommend you grab a girlfriend and agree to do a 30 day challenge together. Also feel free to hashtag me at #freeleethebananagirl so I can follow your progress. I have received many, many testimonials about the positive results of the Raw Till 4 lifestyle, and you will see a number of them in this book. I would also love to hear yours so please feel free to leave them on my Facebook wall.

*You can follow me on:*

 @freeleethebananagirl

 @freeleethebananagirl

 @freeleethebananagirl

 @freeleethebananagirl

## What is the #BananaGirlCleanse?

The BGC is a unique 30 day cleanse to give you a kick start into being the absolute BEST version of yourself. What makes this program so cleansing is the focus on healthy plant foods. Everyone knows that fruits and vegetables are the healthiest, cleanest foods on the planet, so it's about time you go FRUIT yourself and reap the benefits! The diet/lifestyle you will be specifically following is the Raw Till 4 diet which you will soon learn a lot about. Over the next 30 day period, you will probably eat more food than you ever have (and enjoy it!). If you follow the plan correctly, you will feel mentally clear and focused. You will have more energy than ever before and really start to kick ass like a true Banana Girl. The BGC30 includes a basic fitness routine that has helped me shed over 40lbs. There is an epic 30 day Raw Till 4 meal planner with mouth-watering recipes to keep you carbed up and focused. I have a recipe section with over 50 unique mouth-watering recipes. Weekly shopping lists will be included to make the transition smoother and a whole lot more education and fun coming your way. There will be testimonials from other Banana Girls who have cleansed themselves of their disordered eating and now loving life.

## Wait....What IS a BananaGirl?

Although it may sound like you are signing up to some x-rated cult, you are not! You are joining a positive global movement, the Banana Girl Revolution. A movement of carb-strong girls who are standing up against the calorie restrictive diet industry. Girls who are sick of feeling like shit from starvation diets, sick of being lied to and taken advantage of. You may be one of the millions of girls around the World who is suffering from an eating disorder brought about by calorie restrictive diets. Tell me, how many diets have you been on in the past? If your past is anything like mine then more than a few I'm guessing. Now tell me, why aren't you still ON those diets? Why do you keep falling OFF those diets? Why do you feel like crap on those diets? Because that shit don't work sister, that's why. These anti-life diets that recommend you eat/count tiny portions of food (i.e 21 grapes) damage your metabolism, your mental state and teach your body to be a long term fat-storer instead of high performance fat-burner. It's now time to cleanse your colon and renew your vows to your body. Banana Girls are carbed-up and confident, they do not let a number on the scales dictate how they feel about themselves. They are not obsessed with getting skinny at the cost of their health, happiness, and sanity. A banana girl understands healing takes time and recognises how her past of dieting has damaged her body. You are about to join one of the most important movements in the entire world so grab a banana smoothie and lettuce get into this!

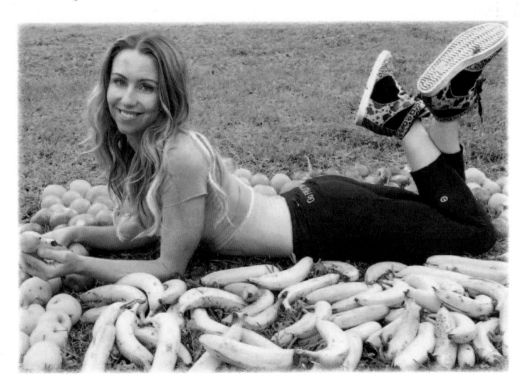

# ONE BANANA GIRLS STORY

*Hey it's Freelee here, and this is my story. I was born in 1980, in Melbourne, Australia, and was raised on a farm in Queensland. We had horses and cows and lots of chickens. We also had our own garden, with easy access to fresh fruit and vegetables. But like almost all Australians, we were clogged up, undercarbed, dehydrated meat and dairy eaters. When I look back, I can see that I always wanted to eat the way I do now; It never felt right - eating my friends. Truth be known like every other person on the planet - I wanted to gobble up all the carbs! There was always a high carb vegan in me, struggling to get out.*

## ONE STORY TAKES ME BACK

When I was young, my family choked down a lot of fish. It was gross. I tried to avoid it like the plague. Yuck. Every night, when we'd sit down to eat, I'd fill my pockets full of tissues, and when mum and dad weren't looking I'd quickly spit-up the fish into the tissues and stuff them back into my pockets. After the meal, I'd sneak off to the bathroom and flush the smelly fish down the toilet. My dirty-little-secret went on for years until my dad finally caught me and gave me the belting of my life! After that, I did what most kids do: I forced that fish down like a well behaved child. It wasn't all crap though. My mum was right into organic fruits and vegetables, and was really trying to get it together. She became my earliest go-to for health. She just didn't have a clue about veganism back then (who did?), so when I was growing up I didn't realize how much cooler and healthier I'd could be if I gave up meat and dairy. I was an active little tacker. There was always a ton of work to be done on the farm, so that kept me busy, but I was also a sprinter in school; I did gymnastics, kick-boxing and even ball-room dancing (yikes!). The push to get off my ass and be active and athletic has always stayed with me, but lettuce be honest - mainly to get skinny.

When I was sixteen I hauled ass from the country straight into the 'big smoke' of Sydney. Coming from the boring hillbilly country, city life was freakin' awesome, but it sucked for my health. I started working at McShit's (yeh McDonald's); and not just working there, but feasting there... a lot! I would eat McShyster's two meals a day, six days a week, and I did that for a full year! Surprised I lived to tell the tale. I put on about 10kgs/22lbs, my skin became a hot mess of oily bumps and my health went down the toilet. Not to mention turning my body into a graveyard for innocent tortured animals.. But, it got even worse.

As you do when you are a naïve country girl; I began dating a drug dealer, and with all the free drugs available, hell no I didn't hold back. I started snacking on ecstacy, speed and cocaine. I became anorexic and bulimic, and dropped nearly 20kg/44lbs in one year! Becoming a skinny bitch was my new full time obsession, regardless of whether I was healthy or not. Even though I was now a walking toothpick with anorexia, it was never skinny enough for me. I could never settle. When girls told me I was getting too skinny I would rub my hands together and think in my head "yeh bitches you just jealous!" and would try to go even further. This period of my life screwed up my health a lot, but one day the shit hit the fan and I finally reached a point where I just couldn't take it anymore.

One of the earliest "kick up the ass" moments came for me in 2001 when I was right into Yoga. At the time I was a sloppy mess but my yoga teacher was vegan and one sexy fit bitch! She also ate bucket loads of raw food. I couldn't ignore how much energy and vibrancy this woman had. Seeing her and hearing about her diet and lifestyle was the "aha!" light bulb mument I needed. I knew I was on to something. I interrogated her about why she looked so good and she just smiled and said "I'm vegan and eat lots of fruits and vegetables" then recommended I buy a juicer. I couldn't order one quick enough and when it arrived it came with a "living foods" recipe book. Even though the recipes weren't all vegan (it actually included raw meat!), it got me to try the raw foods lifestyle. I became obsessed with making little raw food snacks, but nutritionally they were all as fatty as my muffin top, so after a few weeks I "fell off the raw food wagon." For the next five years I rarely thought about raw foods, and continued to be a zombie follower of the latest fad diets. By this stage binging and purging was the norm. I had full fledged bulimia... and no one knew. I became a personal trainer and started hanging out with girls who looked super healthy and fit. We all know the type, young, looks a million bucks but lives on caffeine and junk food. As you know looks can be deceiving: you can rock it on the outside but be killing yourself on the inside. We were all hammering the party drugs and stimulants, most of the guys used steroids regularly. For a little while this seemed to work a treat: girls were complimenting me on how I looked and now I was the one being interrogating on what I was doing. It felt awesome to get that kind of attention and praise, but what they didn't see was that I was dying inside. I wanted their praise because I had no self-esteem of my own.

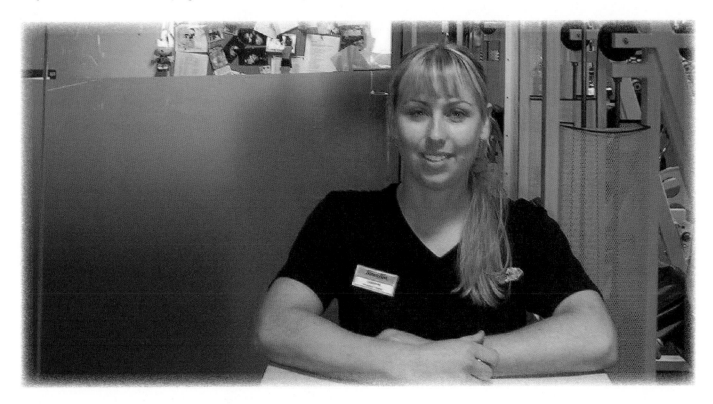

Even though I was a personal trainer, I hardly looked the part and my lifestyle was just straight up unsustainable. I was calorie-restricting and overexercising like a mofo; I was propped up on stimulants and drugs, and my diet was a train wreck. Eventually I "hit the wall" and crashed. I quit my relationship and became a depressed hermit bingeing on anything and everything and then purging. All the weight I had been fighting like crazy to keep off piled right back on again (plus some). I became a systemic candida feeder, and had acne all over my face, shoulders and chest. I felt gross. I had chronic digestive issues with foul explosive diarrhea. My energy was almost completely gone, I felt like a dehydrated sloth on Xanax. Many mornings I couldn't even get my depressed ass out of bed, and would make up excuses to my clients, who I was supposed to be inspiring to health! I was in a hole and suffering from chronic fatigue syndrome. I had reached an all time low, but yet there was still a small fire burning within and it wasn't from poor food combining. I knew in my irritable gut that health needs a more holistic approach and that the body can heal, if I just get out of its way! I knew that if I provided my body with the right conditions, it'll thrive, but like so many girls, I had no freakin' clue where to start.

I started desperately searching for an answer like crazy. I tried the metabolic-type diet, paleo diet, a blood-type diet, atkins, zone, and on and on. Name it, and yep I've probably tried it. But none of them were the answer to my health or tubby weight woes. I began seeing "health professional" doctors, and naturopaths and homeopaths and ayervedics and Chinese medicine practitioners. I wasted thousands of dollars on worthless supplements and "natural therapies." I forked out hundreds of dollars per visit with Australia's leading gastroenterologist, whose only solution was to get me hooked on a new prescription drug. Ugh, I was losing hope. Even though some of them were well-meaning, none of their "solutions" actually worked and they were happy to strip my wallet dry. I didn't want to spend my life "managing" my unhealthy state.

I wanted to get the heck away from drugs and supplements and remedies and snake oil salesman. I just wanted to finally be healthy and look hot in a bikini. Was that too much to ask?

The big changes in my life and my health started in about 2006. First I had gotten myself off recreational drugs and alcohol, and then I took another step and gave up the brain-frying coffee. But I was still far from healthy. After a trip to the Greek islands, where I ate nothing but meaty gut-bloating foods, I came back home feeling like hell. My digestion was worse than ever; so was my skin, and the only thing that was a size zero was my self esteem and bank account. I was regularly suicidal but still clung to a thread of hope and kept pushing forwards. I continued reading and studying nutrition, and eventually came across a magazine article featuring a freakin' gorgeous girl who only ate raw food. She was beautiful and vibrant, and once again the raw food message slapped me in the face, real hard. I had tried raw before and now I wanted more. The raw food movement was pretty dismal at that time, not much was happening so it was challenging to find any books or information on it. I found and read what I could, including books like: "Raw Energy," "The Raw Food Detox Diet," "The Sunfood Diet Success System." There was some ok information, but I wasn't satisfied, so I kept obsessively prowling libraries and book shops for anything I could find.

Next I sniffed out an Aussie raw food forum and typed and typed until my chubby little fingers were suffering from RSI. I was that excited! Yep I felt like I had found the holy grail. That forum experience changed many things in my life. I started blogging and fully committing myself to the raw vegan lifestyle. Go spy on some of my early blogs from this time in my first book: "Go Fruit Yourself!" **www.thebananagirl.com**. You'll see me stuffing up with the same old mistakes every noob makes when coming to the raw food lifestyle: I ate like a sparrow and overexercised, I tried water-feasting, juice-fasting and focused on greens and high fat foods instead of fruits. I did all kinds of crazy stuff because I had NO fully carbed up guidance. I was focused on 100% raw, even without being vegan yet, but still knew diddly squat about how important carbohydrates are in order to be a healthy skinny bitch. I even got confused chefs to make special rice-less sushi for me, so I could eat the raw fish without the carbs! What an undercarbed twit. I kept at it this for a few months, making mistake after mistake, but learning invaluable lessons. Now, when I see other girls coming to the lifestyle, I see them going through the same old painful process. I can feel their frustration and confusion, because I've been there, done that shit!

At the end of 2006 something else happened that would shift my consciousness forever. Although I came to veganism for health and skinny bitch reasons I was suddenly faced with the ethical side of it. One night a friend put on the movie "Earthlings." Suddenly I was hit with a sledgehammer. Had I really had a part in the most gruesome cruel acts imaginable? Heck, it was time to make this right! If you're unsure about veganism, or haven't considered the ethical side, watch Dominion at www.dominionmovement.com.

In January 2007 I became a full fledged vegan, and I've never looked back. I had been educating myself on the in's and out's of diet and nutrition, but didn't know anything about the ethical side. I knew I didn't want to cause suffering to animals, but I had no idea what really happens in order to bring meat and dairy to our frugivorous bellies. After waking up to the evil reality, I began to see the ethical side of veganism, and now this is a big part of my life and why I am vegan. But even going vegan, and even eating raw, didn't 100% improve my health the way I wanted it to. I gained many positives but was still a part time candida-feeder. I knew deep in my colon something wasn't right. Literally. So I kept searching for answers. Then I finally found something sweet and juicy that would help iron out the fatty mistakes I was making. I went to my first ever raw food picnic and met my friend Nadia. While I was inhaling a high-fat gourmet raw creation, she was scoffing only mangoes! Ten delicious, juicy mangoes and nothing else. I was floored. What the heck was this chick thinking? Doesn't she know all the sugar is bad for her? What about candida? What about diabetes?!

I decided I wasn't leaving the picnic without a thorough interrogation of the crazy (yet beautiful) fruit lady in the corner. She happily told me about the high fruit raw vegan lifestyle, she had an intelligent response to everything I threw at her so I was thoroughly fascinated when the picnic broke up. The idea of smashing in endless fruit was far too irresistible for me to ignore so I got home and hit google to research. I joined some random American raw food sites and found out about "Banana Island" and as any sane person does – I proceeded to eat ONLY bananas for almost a month! It was life-changing. During those days I experienced such a drastic shift in my health that I knew this shit was for reals! I had found the answer I had been literally dying to find all these years. Finally I was beginning to understand just how important clean, natural carbs are to be fit, healthy and well just plain awesome! I continued to kick ass on the lifestyle for about 9 months, but then I started starving myself again. I was being an impatient cry baby and wasn't seeing the immediate weight-loss results I wanted to see, and I still thought the answer was to calorie-restrict, so that's what I did and just as the sun is guaranteed to rise each day – I predictably fell off the high fruit lifestyle into high fat cooked vegan foods. I began to binge and stick my fingers down my throat again. To be frank - It was fucking soul destroying. My body knew it needed carbs and was under-fueled, so my calorie starvation led to eat-the-whole-pantry cravings that I just couldn't control (yes girls, those kind of natural cravings for carbs aren't meant to be restricted or controlled!).

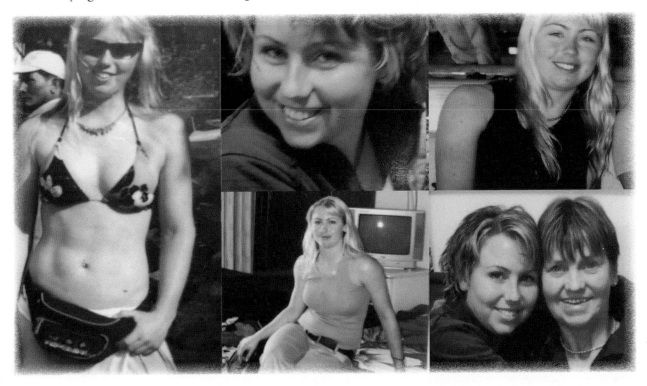

Around then, I went to my second motivational seminar by Tony Robbins, and that did help me get my shit together. I went on a 30-day mango and watermelon challenge with a girlfriend and got myself eyes back on the prize. Tony's techniques helped me stay focused and manifest what I truly wanted in life, not what my ego wanted. After so many years of being a full time bitch to my body I realized that I needed to give it time to heal itself, and that expecting immediate weight-loss results was madness. I actually gained over 20lbs but I started thinking long-term, focusing on getting fit as heck rather than on a superficial thigh gap. When that shift happened, everything started to click.

I finally learned how to do the High Carb Raw Vegan lifestyle the right way: an abundance of fruit, no calorie-restriction mentality, a focus on health, not just on chaffing thighs and belly blubber. My fitness level began to rise. My weight fluctuated for the first few years as my body said "Bitch you gotta pay back the dieting debt!" Yep I had to go through this healing phase after a lengthy past of calorie-restriction and abuse, but then the weight started coming off effortlessly. I've lost about 20 kilos (about 40lbs) in total without ANY calorie-restriction! Now do I have your attention? That's right I said NO calorie restriction. I know you are excited so I promise more about this later in the book. I quit being a part time candida feeder and my skin cleared completely up. Fluffy fruity floaters graced the toilet after years of diarrhea and constipation. My energy went through the roof! And now I am fitter, leaner, happier, and healthier than ever before!

In 2009 I founded the largest, most awesome high carb vegan forum on the web: **www.30bananasaday.com**. Right now there are over 30,000 members and the community is real and supportive. I wanted to spread the good vibes and see happy, healthy fit girls dominate this meaty planet so I started making youtube videos, going to raw-festivals and becoming part of a strong and growing community of healthy, fit, raw vegans.

# GETTING STARTED

## *What is Raw Till 4?*

The first thing you need to know is that Raw Till 4 is a lifestyle (for life), not just a diet, and especially not an overnight quick fix (that doesn't exist). It's a lifestyle, because it includes more than just diet. It includes all the ways we choose to live our lives: diet, exercise, rest, sleep, mental attitude, ethics, etc. With a change towards true health comes true healing, and that is going to include more than just physical changes: it's going to include emotional and mental changes as well. And naturally all those changes will be gradual, not overnight. You gotta be patient girls!

Most girls who start living a RT4 lifestyle find that they begin to see themselves quite differently, with more self-love, more happiness, less self-criticism. They begin to see others differently as well, to see the world differently. Most girls also begin to make ethical connections they had never really considered before, especially those who embrace veganism fully. All these things make RT4 a full lifestyle. It doesn't mean you have to change who you are, what you do for a living, your friends or family, but for most girls the change WILL go beyond just diet. So, what we put in our body is certainly one of the most important aspects of health, but there are many other things to consider as well. Health is wholistic. Healthy body, healthy mind, healthy spirit.

**With that said, here are the key principles to this lifestyle:**

## THE RAW TILL 4 LIFESTYLE: THE BASICS

1. Only plant foods are allowed on this program. No animal products, no exceptions.
2. Raw fruits & greens (mainly fruits) should only be eaten until 4pm (or 2 hours prior to dinner time), then a high carb cooked dinner of high starch plant foods. For best results stick to no cooked food during the day at least 95% of the time.
3. 800+ calories from fruit for breakfast and 800+ from fruit for lunch is recommended for success, then a high carb cooked dinner of 500+ calories. Girls aim for minimum 2100 calories per day, 2400 calories per day to really thrive. Anything below 2100 calories daily is considered a famine by the World Health Organisation which of course I will not ethically recommend.
4. Aim for as close to 90/5/5 as possible in your calorie ratio: that's 90% of calories from carbohydrates and 5% of calories each from fats and proteins. Try to keep fat intake consistently below 10% and carbohydrate intake consistently above 80%. You can work this out easily by punching your numbers in **www.cronometer.com**
5. Stay hydrated! You should pee about 8-12 times per day, and your urine should be clear. Drink 1 litre of water when you wake up in the morning, and 1 litre of water about 30 minutes before each meal for optimal results.
6. Fragmented sodium (salt) should be kept to a minimum. Under 1000mgs per day and under 500mgs for maximum leanness and health. Use herbs, lemon juice, etc. wherever possible in place of salt.
7. Oil is not recommended on this program. It should be kept to an absolute minimum as well. Learn to cook (& eat) without it and you will gain wonderful health benefits. If you go out to dinner where oil is generally unavoidable then ask for less oil.
8. Food should be eaten whole and minimally processed wherever possible. Vegan junk foods, mock meats, tofu and other such foods are not recommended as regular staples but ok occasionally. Minimize these as much as possible for best results.
9. Eat organic wherever possible, it tastes much better and is better for your health and the environment.

10. Try to make one day per week a 100% raw day, I call it #Raw24 in the meal planner. This will help keep the focus on high raw, and will keep your system as clean and optimal as possible.

11. Recommended sources of cooked carbs are: potatoes, root veggies, rice, gluten-free pastas, high carb ancient grains. These should be your main dinner staples, with other wholesome plant-foods as sides.

12. No fruit after cooked food or fermentation and poor digestion will likely result. It can also cause a candida outbreak. If you're still hungry after dinner (or craving sweets) you didn't eat enough fruit during the day for your body's needs. Eat more cooked dinner instead and then aim for more fruit the next day.

13. Big green smoothies are great for getting the calories in for breakfast/lunch. Bananas are a wonderful fruit staple throughout the day. Other high calorie fruits like dates and mangoes make great staples too.

14. Eat unlimited calories at every meal, no restriction. The majority of your calories each day should come from fruit. Don't under eat on fruit during the day or "save up" your calories for dinner time. RT4 is about abundance at every meal.

15. Chickpeas, beans, lentils are not high carb choices so should be used as side dishes instead of main staples.

16. Move your body daily. Find an activity you love and make it your playful exercise. Exercise is critical to overall health and well-being; it stimulates your metabolism and gets everything flowing well. Plus it's great for our mood! Building up a regular sweat will promote optimal health results on this lifestyle.

17. Make sure to get lots of rest, relaxation and good sleep. Learning to incorporate good rest, early nights, and regular sleeping patterns into your life will greatly improve your overall health.

18. Be sure to get some sun. Full body sunbathing is recommended, for a minimum of 20 minutes every day. Get in your vitamin D and boost your sense of well-being.

19. If necessary, supplement B-12 with either shots or sublinguals. Around 40% of the population (vegan or not) are B12 deficient, and this can greatly reduce our health results.

20. Practice gratitude and peaceful emotions at meal time, and get a vision book started! Be sure to enjoy this journey. Focus on long-term health instead of short-term results. This is a lifestyle you can rock for the rest of your life, and if you focus on becoming healthy inside, in time you'll then end up looking healthy and hot on the outside. You will come to a healthy weight naturally if you give your body a good foundation of healthy habits. Consistency and patience are key!

## Why Plant-Foods Only?

This is the most important thing you can do for your health, and for the health of the planet. Until you give up all animal products, you'll never become the fittest, healthiest, happiest version of yourself. This is just a small selection; the reasons are endless. Going vegan is the first step towards a healthy, happy, rewarding life, and the first step towards solving some of the world's most important problems.

### A few reasons to avoid animal flesh ("meat"), secretions ("dairy") and menses ("eggs"):

1. Animal products create an acidic environment in the body, leading to severe health issues, like osteoporosis.
2. All animal products are high in fat and cholesterol, which clog the arteries and are the number one cause of heart disease.
3. Animal protein causes increased cancer-cell production, and is one of the leading causes of the human cancer epidemic.
4. Animal fat impedes the work of insulin, leading to blood-sugar issues and ultimately to diabetes.
5. The fat you eat is the fat you wear: animal fats are easily stored by the body, and are the number one reason behind the obesity epidemic.
6. Animal agriculture is the most environmentally damaging industry in the world according to the United Nations.
7. Animal products are loaded with hormones and anti-biotics that aren't meant to be in your body and cause a variety of serious health issues.
8. Killing animals for food is unnecessary and cruel. Most farmed animals live lives of suffering we can't even imagine.

# THE ETHICAL SIDE OF NOT EATING ANIMALS

One thing I see too often in the vegan movement is girls under eating on carbohydrates and going back to eating their animal friends. I came to a high carb, raw vegan lifestyle straight from eating diced and sliced animals. I didn't develop the ethical vegan side until about 6 months into following this lifestyle. I simply didn't educate myself as to what was involved in the production of animal products.

I knew I didn't want to cause anymore suffering to animals but was never exposed to what really happened in those massive concentration camps called slaughterhouses. That was until I watched the truth on youtube, I made myself watch slaughterhouse videos. You may think that's crazy but what I think is crazier is not knowing where my food is from. It changed my consciousness forever. If you are serious about knowing the whole truth about the origin of what you consume (or previously consumed) then you owe it to yourself and the animals to watch the "Best Speech You Will Ever Hear" by Gary Yourofsky on YouTube. Please prioritize this. It is bound to have a positive effect on your future food choices and health. Over the years, I have educated myself not only on the damage animal products inflict on the body but also about the torture, slaughter, and rape associated with the consumption of all animal products. To be successful on the Raw Till 4 path, you must be on this lifestyle for worthwhile reasons, wanting to lose fat off your thighs or belly alone is NOT a worthwhile reason and will always eventually lead to the wrong foods. Increasing health and vitality and at the same time wanting to make this world a better place for all who inhabit it, ARE worthwhile reasons.

## But isn't a Vegetarian diet less cruel?

Many say that the industry associated with the promotion and production of dairy and eggs is even crueler than the ones dealing directly with the slaughter and sale of flesh. Cows and chickens are abused (including routinely raped) for longer periods and inevitably slaughtered when their productivity declines (at about a 5th of their natural lifespan). Everyone eats animals in our society right? It must be ok then...? Wrong. Wrong is wrong even if everyone is doing it, right is right even if nobody is doing it.

I grew up with cows, let me tell you, they are the most beautiful, gentle giants you may ever meet. Sometimes one of 'our' cows (we called her Missy) would let me drape my body across her back in the sun while she gorged on the grass. She was so patient and kind. One of the calves she had was like a best friend to me. We would play for hours. She would head-butt me playfully and spring around happily like a puppy dog. Anyone who has ever closely associated with calves will likely relay a similar experience. I will always cherish those days.

In the dairies (yes organic grass-fed as well) cows just like Missy have their calves ripped away from them at birth and often slaughtered immediately or sold to the veal industry. After spending months being permanently confined to a box in which they cannot ever turn, the calves bodies are ground up at the rendering plant where they are often fed back to other cows and even to their mothers. These are herbivorous, feeling, animals folks! We have turned these gentle giants into unwilling carnivores (& even cannibals). The reason this is done is because the cholesterol content of the dismembered animal mix increases milk production. The industry call it "enriched" feed - enriched with a mix of animal body parts, road kill, euthanized dogs and cats, fish then cooked ground up and mixed with grains. The only reason the cannibalism may be stopped is due to the outbreak of mad cow disease.

**Jeanie Williams**  6 hours ago
Freelee, I love you and I love your message. I wish I would have found you when I was much younger (you weren't born yet)! I spent over 30 years yo yo dieting and OBSESSING about every damn thing that went in my mouth. I was never happy with how I looked. I wasted precious time on this. Time I should have spent doing other things more important. Young women, please listen to Freelee. Nothing, I mean nothing works out there in the "diet" world. It is all crap feeding on our insecurities. People are making millions of dollars off of us and it is stupid. I was a vegetarian, and then a vegan and I am now RT4. (My profile pic shows me with a glass of wine. I don't do that anymore! I feel amazing and am losing weight and eating and eating and eating. I have more energy than I did in my 20s. Thank you!!!!!!!!!!!!!!!!!
Show less

1 👍 👎

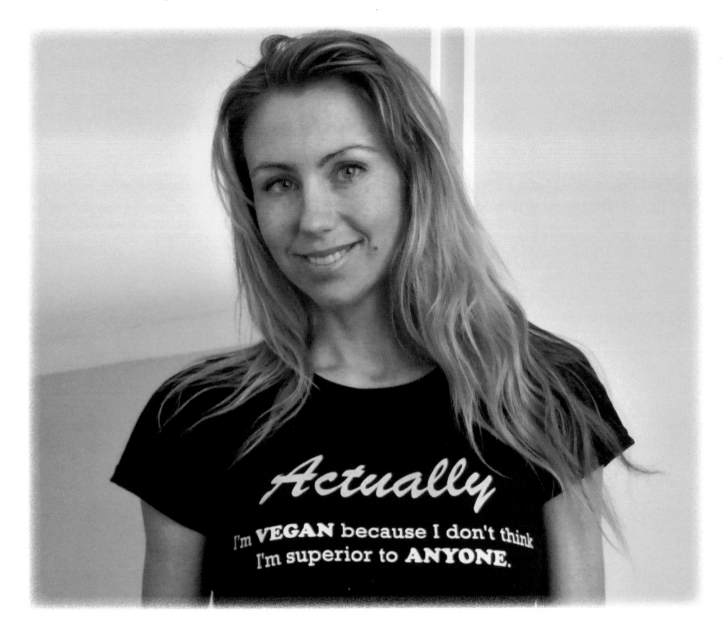

**Here is a relevant quote from Will Tuttle out of his amazing book 'The World Peace Diet':**

*"Of all the mammals, it is the cow whose maternal instinct has been perhaps the most obvious and celebrated. Her gentle and patient eyes, her natural mothering way with her calf, licking, feeding and watching over her baby and her loud lamenting when the calf is taken away from her...She cannot fight the hands that steal her offspring away or speak to us in human words, telling us how deeply it hurts her but it is obvious to anyone with eyes to see and ears to hear, for us to ignore her suffering and the suffering of her calf, hundreds, thousands, millions of times over, is to ignore and deny our own decency. There is a deep and terrible transgression in this. The unnatural coveting of the calf's mothers milk several thousand years ago and the building of a whole culture around the stealing of milk, the killing of the mother and her children and justifying the whole horrific thing by mythologizing it – the Lord promising us the land of milk and honey. This violent theft of milk from enslaved mothers planted seeds of war and exploitation that are tragically almost completely invisible. Today our culture takes milk for granted, it is aggressively promoted around the world. How can we ever hope for peace when we practice such shameful violence on such a massive scale"*

There really is no other reality to it - When we consume milk products from ANY mammals (especially as females), we initiate the rape, exploitation and death of other female animals. It's time to wake up to the enormity of consuming animal products. It's time to think for ourselves and ask our heart what is the right thing to do.

**For more information please visit this website by Gary Yourofsky:** www.adaptt.org

# FRUIT YOURSELF!
# (MAJORITY OF CALS FROM FRUIT)

Raw fruit is our ideal food, and it's the best thing you can possibly live on during the day. On RT4, you want the majority of your calories to come from whole, fresh, ripe, raw (preferably organic) fruit! Not only will this give you all the nutrition your body needs, it'll also keep you hydrated, give you amazingly healthy skin, help you burn fat and make you a lean, mean fruit-muncher for life!

Getting into a good morning routine is so important on this lifestyle. After we've been sleeping for 8 or more hours (see the section on sleep), our bodies are ready for two things: hydration and fuel! I highly recommend drinking between 500ml and 1 litre of water when you get up in the morning. It'll set your day up well and give you a hydration boost. Try to leave a bit of time before drinking the water and having breakfast: your body will absorb the water more quickly and easily if it's not accompanied by food. I'll often go outside, maybe for a short run or bike-ride: get the body moving and the blood flowing to kick-start the day. Then I'll have my big breakfast.

Remember, RT4 isn't the kind of strict lifestyle that demands you to schedule every meal and workout perfectly; the key is to learn the principles and then make the diet work in your life. Some people start work bright and early in the morning; some can wake up and take their time; some have to help get their kids off to school. So the morning principles are: 1) initial hydration; 2) move your body a bit if you have the time; and 3) a big fruity-meal. You can work that into your schedule however you can.

Your breakfast really should be a minimum of 800 calories. Most long-term successful high carb vegans make breakfast the biggest meal of the day. It really gets your body and brain functioning top-notch if you can fuel yourself up early in the day. Smoothies are my preferred breakfast, and most people find it much easier to eat a high-calorie fruit meal in the morning if it's done as a smoothy. Check out the recipes section for some absofruitly delicious smoothy recipes!

Once you've had your high-calorie, high-carb fruity breakfast, you'll be good to go for a few hours. Some people like to graze during the day, and that's fine, but I recommend focusing on meals rather than constant snacking. Focusing on meals and keeping the number of ingredients used in each meal to a minimum, will help you optimise your digestion. Monomeals are the best for digestion, so if you find you're having any kinds of digestion issues when first coming to the lifestyle, try making the first two meals of the day monomeals. My first two meals of the day are most often monomeals.

As lunch gets closer, make sure you've been staying hydrated and peeing clear. It's a good habit to get into to drink another litre of water about a half-hour before your lunch meal as well, just to keep you hydrated and to set yourself up for easy digestion. For lunch you want to have another big fruity meal, again aim for a minimum of 800 calories. This is the meal where most of us like to really savour some whole fruits in their natural form. You can make mono meals from melons (honeydew, cantaloupe, watermelon) if you've got the stomach capacity to get in enough carbs; or you can make a meal of whole bananas with whole dates; or maybe a plate of persimmons or mangoes or grapes or other mouth-watering sweet fruits! There are so many fruits to choose from, so pick what you love, and what you can seasonally find, and fill up to your heart's content!

Making another smoothy for lunch is also a good option, especially for those with busier lives. You can make an additional smoothy in the morning and take it to work with you also (though if you do, be careful not to oxidise the fruit too much when blending, and be sure to seal the container with no air inside). For those of you who work in an office, you might be able to bring fruit and make a smoothie at work. The key is to load up on the fruity-carbs. By the time you're done lunch, ideally you should've eaten a minimum of 1500 calories, so your body and mind will be full of energy and you'll be able to easily wait until dinner without hunger and cravings. If you're craving anything after lunch, it means you haven't eaten enough. The fruit meals are the center focus of this lifestyle. That's where you want most of your calories to come from, and that's where you'll get the majority of your nutritional value. So don't hold back; aim for big fruity meals and eat up those carbs! Everyone has their favourite fruits, and there are literally hundreds of varieties of fruit in the world. Not all fruits are as calorically-dense as others though (which is one reason bananas and dates are so popular on this lifestyle), so it pays to know how many cals you're getting from each fruit. Here's a little table of some common fruits, showing the calorie-densities and macronutrient breakdown (of course, each fruit also has its own unique nutritional values). This list isn't extensive, but it'll give you a basic starting point.

After that, go out and explore all the wonderful and exotic fruits Mother Earth gives us! :)

| Fruit | Cals/100g | Carbs % | Fat % | Protein % |
|---|---|---|---|---|
| Dates | 280 | 98 | 0 | 2 |
| Persimmons | 130 | 95 | 3 | 2 |
| Jackfruit | 100 | 92 | 3 | 5 |
| Bananas | 90 | 93 | 3 | 4 |
| Grapes | 70 | 94 | 2 | 4 |
| Mangoes | 60 | 94 | 3 | 3 |
| Pears | 60 | 96 | 2 | 2 |
| Blueberries | 60 | 91 | 5 | 4 |
| Oranges | 50 | 91 | 2 | 7 |
| Apples | 50 | 95 | 3 | 2 |
| Plums (mixed, avg.) | 50 | 90 | 5 | 5 |
| Raspberries | 50 | 82 | 10 | 8 |
| Peaches | 40 | 87 | 5 | 8 |
| Papayas | 40 | 92 | 3 | 5 |
| Honeydew Melon | 40 | 92 | 3 | 5 |
| Cantaloupe | 30 | 87 | 5 | 8 |
| Watermelon | 30 | 89 | 4 | 7 |
| Strawberries | 30 | 85 | 8 | 7 |
| Durian* | 150 | 67 | 30 | 3 |
| Avocado* | 160 | 19 | 77 | 4 |

*Some fruits are high in calories, but also high in fat, so shouldn't be eaten every day or in big quantities. They are delicious though.

**Mello Pokemaster**  23 minutes ago

I've only been on raw till four for a week and other than being a little bloated after a meal i feel absolutely amazing. I've had a past of both bulimia and anorexia, i also used to use shit tons of laxatives and counted everything I ate, but now that I'm on raw till four I've noticed I'm starting to care less and less about eating too much and I actually feel proud when i look and see I've eaten 2500+ calories in a day. I honestly feel so lucky to have stumbled across freelees channel and for so long i was always back and forth with not wanting to do raw till 4 and wanting to do it but being too scared to start. I'm so proud of myself to have started this long healing journey that my body so desperately needs and I know I'm gonna enjoy everyday for the rest of my life because of raw till 4. Thank you soooooooooo much freelee and durianrider for expressing your love and respect for this lifestyle.
Show less

👍 👎

# ROOT YOURSELF!
# (HIGH-CARB COOKED DINNER)

After filling up on fruit during the day, you can then have a nice, nutritious and delicious cooked vegan meal for dinner. Use rice, sweet or regular potatoes, root vegetables, etc., to make up the majority of the calories in your dinner. Chickpeas, beans, lentils, etc., are not high carb foods, so don't make them main staples. If you want, just have them as a side dish. Focus on high carbs, low fat, low protein (and use cronometer or a similar program until you get used to identifying high-carb foods).

Add a big, green, leafy salad to top it all off. Leafy greens will help with digestion, give you lots of important vitamins and minerals and buffer any acidity from cooked foods. Get creative, mix it up, try new recipes, and create easy-to-make, mouth-watering homemade dressings (lowfat, of course!).

For dinner, it works well to aim for 500 calories or more as a target. If you've had big, high-carb meals for breakfast and lunch you can probably meet your 2100 minimum with a smaller cooked dinner, but remember: 2100 is the minimum, so don't feel any need to stop there. I don't. I often eat over 3000 calories a day. Most girls will feel best on 2400 or more calories per day (even small and lean women), especially if you're enjoying getting outside and moving your body every day. If you've had a particularly intense exercise day, make sure to really get the calories in. Your body will be starving for them, so when it asks for more carbs, give them to it.

Also: avoid eating sweet fruits, sugars, etc., after the cooked dinner. They tend to get blocked by the cooked food and may ferment in your gut instead of digesting quickly, as sugars are meant to do. Once you transition from raw to cooked during the day, stick with cooked from then on. This is the main reason the cooked meal is set up to be the last one of the day: it'll be the slowest digesting meal. Fruit digests faster than any other food (which is natural, since it's the food we're designed for), while cooked plant-foods digest much slower. Having the cooked meal at the end of the day means you're allowing it all night to digest. By the time you wake up to have a morning smoothy, the cooked meal will be done and gone.

Here are a few examples of high-carb foods, listed by their macro-nutrient ratios. The primary high-carb foods are the ones that should make up the main source of calories in any cooked RT4 meal: they're both high-carb and calorie-dense. The secondary foods (either of lower carb ratio or lower calorie-density) can be used for side-dishes, sauces, soups, etc..

Note: use resources like: cronometer.com, nutritiondata.self.com, etc., to learn about the nutritional values of each food.

| Primary Cooked Foods | Carbs % | Fat % | Protein % |
|---|---|---|---|
| Rice (brown) | 86 | 7 | 7 |
| Rice (white) | 91 | 2 | 7 |
| Potatoes (mixed, avg.) | 90 | 2 | 8 |
| Yams | 95 | 1 | 4 |
| Sweet Potatoes | 93 | 2 | 5 |
| Corn (pasta, couscous, etc) | 90 | 5 | 5 |
| Cassava | 97 | 1 | 2 |

A wide variety of lightly cooked (steamed/boiled) vegetables make for wonderful side-dishes. Certain fruits, like mangoes, dates, etc., can be used in cooking sauces, but generally fruit doesn't combine well with cooked food. Check out the recipes section for examples and ideas of high-carb cooked dinners!

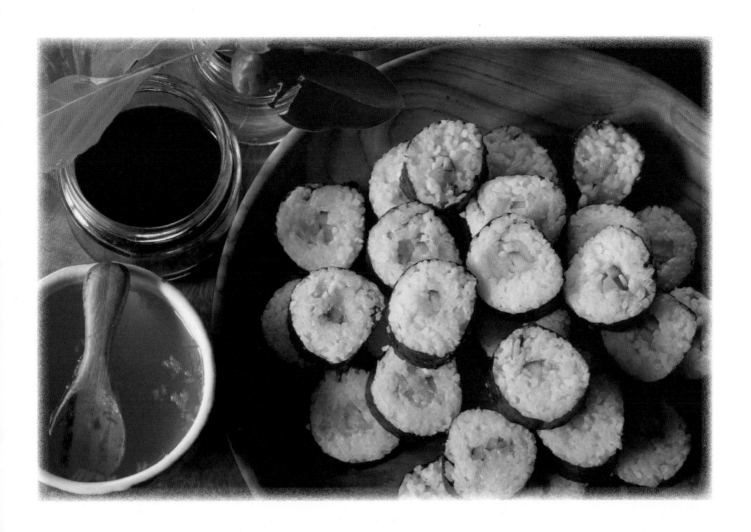

| Secondary Cooked Foods | Carbs % | Fat % | Protein % |
|---|---|---|---|
| Squash (butternut, acorn) | 92 | 5 | 2 |
| Squash (spaghetti) | 86 | 8 | 6 |
| Pumpkin | 88 | 3 | 9 |
| Beets | 86 | 3 | 11 |
| Rutabagas | 86 | 5 | 9 |
| Parsnips | 91 | 4 | 5 |
| Eggplant | 89 | 5 | 6 |
| Quinoa | 72 | 14 | 14 |
| Beans (mixed, avg.) | 70-80 | 3-7 | 14-24 |
| Lentils | 70 | 4 | 26 |
| Chickpeas (garbanzos) | 68 | 13 | 19 |

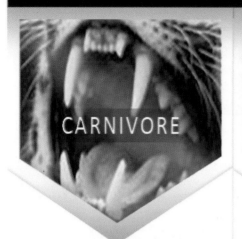
## CARNIVORE

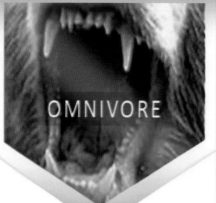
## OMNIVORE

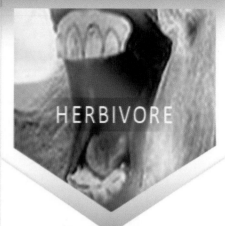
## HERBIVORE

| CARNIVORE | OMNIVORE | HERBIVORE |
| --- | --- | --- |
| Physiological food : meat | PF : meat & vegetables | PF : grass & tree foliage |
| 4 paws with claws | 4 paws with claws/hooves | 4 paws with hooves |
| Walks on 4 paws | Walks on 4 paws | Walks on 4 paws |
| Mouth opening : large | Mouth opening : large | Mouth opening : small |
| Great sharp fangs | Great sharp fangs | Rudimentary, blunt canines |
| Short and pointed incisors | Short and pointed incisors | Big and flattened incisors |
| Blade shaped molars | Blade shaped/crushing molars | Flattened & strong molars |
| Lower jaw embedded inside of the top; no lateral or forward mobility | Lower jaw embedded inside of the top; no lateral or forward mobility/minimal | Upper jaw sits on the bottom; great lateral and forward mobility |
| Shear; swallow w/o chewing | Shear & swallow/crushing | No shear; chew much |
| Small salivary glands | Small salivary glands | Big salivary glands |
| Acid saliva without ptyallin | Acid saliva without ptyallin | Alkaline saliva with ptyallin |
| Acid urine | Acid urine | Alkaline urine |
| Renal secretion of uricase | Renal secretion of uricase | Does not secrete uricase |
| Strong hydrochloric acid | Strong hydrochloric acid | Weak hydrochloric acid |
| Does not requires fiber to stimulate peristalsis | Does not requires fiber to stimulate peristalsis | Requires fiber to stimulate peristalsis |
| Metabolize large amount of cholesterol and vitamin A | Metabolize large amount of cholesterol and vitamin A | Metabolize small amount of cholesterol and vitamin A |
| Sweat glands in the paws; gasp to cool the blood | Sweat glands in the whole body | Sweat glands in the whole body |
| Intestine from 1.5 to 3 times body length | Intestine 3 times body length | Intestine 20 times body length |
| Colon short smooth alkaline | Colon short smooth alkaline | Colon long complex acid |
| Not metabolize cellulose | Not metabolize cellulose | Metabolize cellulose |
| Complete digestion 2-4 hrs | Complete digestion 6-10 hrs | Complete digestion 24-48 hrs |

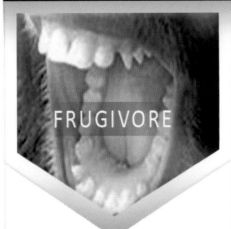

FRUGIVORE

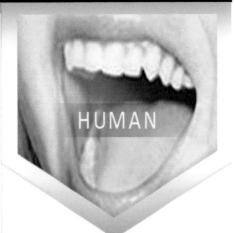

HUMAN

| FRUGIVORE | HUMAN |
| --- | --- |
| PF : fruits, vegetables, nuts | PF : fruits, vegetables, nuts |
| Prehensile hands and feet | Prehensile hands |
| Walks on 4 paws/upright | Walks upright |
| Mouth opening : small/M | Mouth opening : small |
| Canines for defense | Rudimentary, blunt canines |
| Big and flattened incisors | Big and flattened incisors |
| Flattened molars | Flattened molars |
| Upper jaw sits on the bottom; great lateral and forward mobility | Upper jaw sits on the bottom; great lateral and forward mobility |
| No shear; chew their food | No shear; chew their food |
| Big salivary glands | Big salivary glands |
| Alkaline saliva with ptyallin | Alkaline saliva with ptyallin |
| Alkaline urine | Alkaline urine |
| Does not secrete uricase | Does not secrete uricase |
| Weak hydrochloric acid | Weak hydrochloric acid |
| Requires fiber to stimulate peristalsis | Requires fiber to stimulate peristalsis |
| Metabolize small amount of cholesterol and vitamin A | Metabolize small amount of cholesterol and vitamin A |
| Sweat glands in the whole body | Sweat glands in the whole body |
| Intestine 9 times body length | Intestine 9 times body length |
| Colon long sacculated acid | Colon long sacculated acid |
| Does not metabolize cellulose | Does not metabolize cellulose |
| Complete digestion 12-18 hrs | Complete digestion 12-18 hrs |

# #RAW24

During the 30 day BGC, there are 4 all-raw days included. This will help you keep the goal to be as raw as possible, and can be a nice mix in the week. You can set a certain day of the week if you want, say, Raw Mondays maybe. It's something to have fun with, but not something to really pressure yourself about. It can be easy to slide into a routine where we start getting most of our calories from our cooked dinners, with less and less from our raw breakfasts and lunches, so aiming to have one day a week when you forego the cooked dinner in favour of a big plate of fruit or a giant salad, or a delicious smoothie, or other raw creations, can really help build up the habit of making fruit the priority. If you find yourself sliding into that kind of routine, go Raw24 to set yourself back on track.

## How does RT4 compare to the McDougall plan?

The basic foundation is the same, and both diets are based on the same nutritional science. The main difference is that RT4 focus on high calorie raw fruit meals during the day, while Dr. McDougall recommends focusing on starches (though he also wants girls to include "a plentiful supply of fruits and vegetables"). I also focus more on abundant calories, while many who do the McDougall plan will restrict their calories for weight loss, or generally eat less than I would recommend. I cannot say that the diets are the same, but in my view, their similarities far outweigh their differences.

# ABOUT THE RT4 PRINCIPLES

## Why is there a calorie minimum, and isn't that too many calories?!

The number one reason girls fail on the high carb vegan/Raw Till 4 lifestyle is that they undereat. They "listen to their body" or "listen for true hunger" and eat only until they "feel full," but they simply don't get enough fuel for their body and eventually their body just takes over and their cravings overwhelm them. Next thing you know, they're going out for a steak dinner and ranting about how the vegan lifestyle didn't work for them! I believe in objective calculated standards for our health because subjective standards just aren't trustworthy. I don't believe in listening to your body at the early stage on this lifestyle, especially when your body is in a state of healing or ill-health after years of dieting. Someone who has been calorie restricting for most of their life might "feel full" after 3 bananas. Does that mean they only need 3 bananas per meal to thrive, is that what they're body is telling them? Of course not. They need the same number of calories from healthy sources as any other active adult. But their body's signals are messed up and aren't truly telling them what they need. They need to re-train their body signals by focusing on objective goals. This is how anorexia is treated in treatment centers, for instance. They don't listen to the patient's body and base how much they eat on that. No, they set an objective target and the patients force themselves to meet it until it begins to feel natural and their health begins to return. The same idea applies to anyone coming from an unhealthy background: they need clear objective goals to aim for in order to re-train their body into healthy habits. We cannot just trust our old unhealthy habits to somehow bring us to a state of health. Girls, we need to REPROGRAM ourselves for health, from the inside out.

Over the years, I have refined my approach to be the most helpful and objective as I can based on observing and coaching thousands of girls and based on my own long-term experience with the lifestyle. I have come to recommend a bare minimum of 2100 calories for women. Less than 2100 calories per day for ANY women over time is almost guaranteed to develop vitamin and mineral deficiencies (particularly as the quality of conventional fruit, veggies and grains isn't as good as it could be), and definitely guaranteed to develop an energy deficiency for any active adult life. The World Health Organisation states that anything below 2100 calories per day is famine/starvation and recommending anything below that would be unethical, immoral and just darn unhelpful! I find again and again and again that those girls who consistently meet the calorie minimum kick arse on the lifestyle long term, while those who don't end up struggling or give up altogether and fall back into their old diet yoyo, often going all the way back to killing our animal friends for food.

It's also important to know that it's completely natural to have a full, round "buddha" belly after eating a meal. That may feel over-stuffed to a newbie, but over time it'll feel normal, because our stomachs are designed to be able to stretch that way. If you've eaten standard processed foods and animal products for most of your life (like most of us had before coming to the lifestyle) then your stomach will be used to getting lots of calories in a small volume of food. When you switch to a plant-based diet you'll need to eat much more volume in order to get the same number of calories. So you'll need to re-train your stomach to stretch enough to get the calories you need to thrive. It may feel difficult in the first few days or weeks, but in time it'll feel natural and easy to eat 2100+ calories from fruit and starches every day! When that happens, you'll be set up to thrive for the rest of your life.

To demonstrate that my calorie recommendations aren't invented or out of touch with the scientifically demonstrated needs of adults, here are the recommendations for healthy, active adults drawn from the "Dietary Guidelines for Americans". These numbers are for "a lifestyle that includes physical activity equivalent to walking more than 3 miles per day at 3 to 4 miles per hour, in addition to the light physical activity associated with typical day-to-day life." In other words, the basic life of an average adult. Anyone with increased physical activity, sports training, etc., is going to need more calories to fuel their athletic life. With RT4, I recognise the importance of fitness for overall health, and I also recognise that even when I go well over these numbers I remain lean long term because I am keeping my fat intake low and my carbohydrate intake high (and carbs don't make you fat).

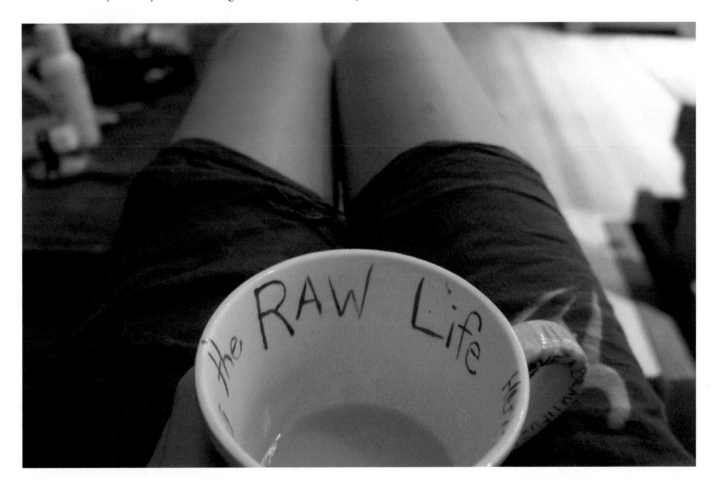

| Gender | Age (Years) | Calories Required |
|---|---|---|
| Child | 2-3 | 1,000 - 1,400 |
| Female | 4-8 | 1,400 - 1,800 |
| Female | 9-13 | 1,800 - 2,200 |
| Female | 14-18 | 2,400 |
| Female | 19-30 | 2,400 |
| Female | 31-50 | 2,200 |
| Female | 51+ | 2,100 - 2,200 |
| Male | 4-8 | 1,600 - 2,000 |
| Male | 9-13 | 2,000 - 2,600 |
| Male | 14-18 | 2,800 - 3,200 |
| Male | 19-30 | 3,000 |
| Male | 31-50 | 2,800 - 3,000 |
| Male | 51+ | 2,400 - 2,800 |

**Estimated Calorie Needs Per Day**

So you can see that abundant calories are essential to our health and well-being, and that having an objective number is critical to long-term success. Remember: Carb up to kick arse! Don't shy away from abundant calories from clean, healthy fruits, starches and veggies! For anyone still concerned about excess carbohydrate calories turning into fat, take it from one of the most well educated doctors on the planet, who has spent his life specialising in the health benefits of a carbohydrate (largely starch) based diet: **Excess Starch Does Not Turn to Body Fat.**

*"A widely held belief is that the sugars in starches are readily converted into fat and then stored unattractively in the abdomen, hips, and buttock. Incorrect! And there is no disagreement about the truth among scientists or their published scientific research. After eating, the complex carbohydrates found in starches, such as rice, are digested into simple sugars in the intestine and then absorbed into the bloodstream where they are transported to trillions of cells in the body in order to provide for energy. Carbohydrates (sugars) consumed in excess of the body's daily needs can be stored (invisibly) as glycogen in the muscles and liver. The total storage capacity for glycogen is about two pounds. Carbohydrates consumed in excess of our need and beyond our limited storage capacity are not readily stored as body fat. Instead, these excess carbohydrate calories are burned off as heat (a process known as facultative dietary thermogenesis) or used in physical movements not associated with exercise.*

*The process of turning sugars into fats is known as de novo lipogenesis. Some animals, such as pigs and cows, can efficiently convert the low-energy, inexpensive carbohydrates found in grains and grasses into calorie-dense fats. This metabolic efficiency makes pigs and cows ideal "food animals." Bees also perform de novo lipogenesis; converting honey (simple carbohydrates) into wax (fats). However, human beings are very inefficient at this process and as a result de novo lipogenesis does not occur under usual living conditions in girls. When, during extreme conditions, de novo lipogenesis does occur the metabolic cost is about 30% of the calories consumed—a very wasteful process. Under experimental laboratory conditions overfeeding of large amounts of simple sugars to subjects will result in a little bit of de novo lipogenesis. For example, trim and obese girls were overfed 50% more total calories than they usually ate in a day, along with an extra 3.5 ounces (135 grams) of refined sugar.*

*From this overfeeding the girls produced less than 4 grams (36 calories) of fat daily, which means a person would have to be overfed by this amount of extra calories and sugar every day for nearly 4 months in order to gain one extra pound of body fat. Obviously, even overeating substantial quantities of refined and processed carbohydrates is a relatively unimportant source of body fat. So where does all that belly fat come from? The fat you eat is the fat you wear.*"—Dr. John McDougall, "People Passionate about Starches are Healthy and Beautiful," March, 2009.

## *Is it ok to fast or juice feast on this lifestyle?*

Heck. No. I don't recommend fasting or juice-fasting/feasting on this lifestyle. It's ok to have some juice during the day, especially if you can fresh-squeeze it yourself, but going on a juice fast is terrible for your health and potentially damages your metabolism and digestion. Fasting is starvation. It puts your body into a state of restriction and turns you into a chubby fat-storer. You might lose some initial weight by fasting or juice-feasting—it's easy to lose weight by starving ourselves—but as soon as you try to return to your normal eating habits you'll gain it all back and more. Then what do girls do? Another fast, or another juice feast to "cleanse" or drop the weight again. I see it time and time again. It's a yoyo game, and it's not one you want to play. Focus on long term consistency. Get all the calories and nutrients you need daily; exercise daily; create sustainable habits, and over time your body will find health and balance and you'll get all the results you've ever dreamed of. Fasting and juice-feasting are shortcuts that simply don't work.

Here's something to consider: have you ever wondered why some so-called diet gurus are constantly "detoxing," juice-fasting or water-fasting because they feel they need to "cleanse" their system? If your diet and lifestyle are truly healthy and sustainable, like RT4 is, there's no need to continually detox or cleanse all the time. The unending need to "detox" or "cleanse" is a sure sign that someone's diet/lifestyle plan isn't truly healthy or sustainable. Those who are consistently healthy long term don't detox or cleanse; they don't need to, because they're not building up toxins or collecting junk in their digestive system. And that's the goal with RT4: consistent health, day in and day out, for the rest of your life.

**On Juicing:**
https://www.30bananasaday.com/profiles/blogs/juicingsideeffects
https://youtu.be/Ihq93daJMc0
https://www.facebook.com/TheBananaGirl/posts/553409958059627

**On the importance of fiber:**
https://nutritionfacts.org/topics/fiber/
https://pcrm.org/health/cancer-resources/diet-cancer/nutrition/how-fiber-helps-protect-against-cancer
https://nutritionfacts.org/video/fiber-vs-breast-cancer/
https://www.drmcdougall.com/health/education/health-science/featured-articles/articles/fiber-reduces-heart-attack-risk/
https://www.ncbi.nlm.nih.gov/pubmed/7616842
https://care.diabetesjournals.org/content/20/4/545.abstract

**Jasmine Hana McKittens** This lifestyle has helped my eating disorder, a disorder I nearly died from. I was going days without anything but diet coke, and then would have this huge binge feast of fries, donuts, cakes etc. I would eat stuff I didn't even like just because it was food! Now I eat every day all day, and binge on bananas and dates! There's nothing more exciting then waking up to a banana smoothie and having curry and rice for dinner, and I never feel fat and ugly anymore.
Unlike · Reply · 👍 16 · 12 hrs

**Freelee the Banana Girl** ✓ Just so cool to hear this 😊
Like · Commented on by Freelee Bell [?] · Just now

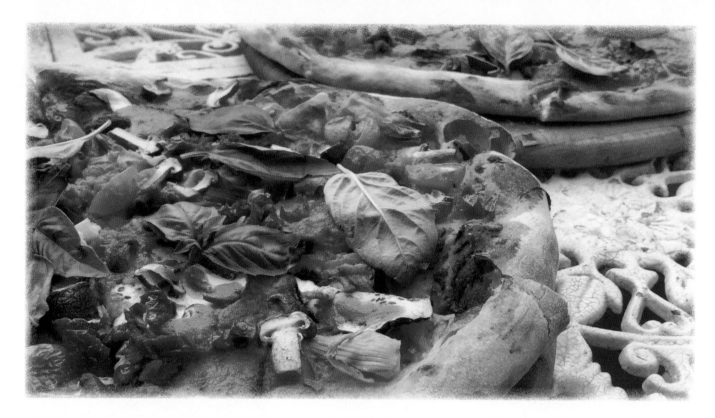

## Do I have to wait until exactly 4pm to eat cooked food?

No girlfriend, you don't. RT4 isn't the kind of diet plan that is so strict. The idea is to eat raw until a couple of hours before our cooked dinner (to give the raw fruit enough time to move through our stomach). For most girls this will be around 4pm, and that's where the name of the lifestyle comes from, but you can customize the principles of RT4 to suit your life. Everyone has a unique life-situation and a unique schedule, so try to adapt the lifestyle as best you can to fit the life you want to live. Stick to fruits for your first two meals of the day, and try to get the majority of your calories for the day from those raw fruits. Then switch to a cooked meal to finish the day. Once you've switched to a cooked meal, stay on cooked food for the rest of the day. Easy peasy!

## Can I eat cooked for lunch too?

Yes, it's ok once and a while, but it's better not to make a regular habit of it—always try to fill up on fruit as much as you can. I understand that some days it might be too much of an inconvenience to have a raw lunch (maybe you have a business meeting or just have no access to ripe fruit, etc.). On those days it's fine to have a high carb cooked lunch and then another high carb cooked dinner. People are regularly treating and reversing our society's main diseases through a carbohydrate focused plant-based diet, whether cooked or raw, so if you're not able to go as high-raw as some others, that's fine: you'll still be eating one of the healthiest diets on the planet! For optimal results on RT4, especially in the beginning, I do recommend always trying to get the majority of calories from fruit, day in and day out. But I realize that you live in the real world, so just do YOUR best.

## Why can't I eat fruit after cooked food?

Raw fruit digests much faster than cooked starches. Eating raw fruits before cooked starches works perfectly because the fruit can digest quickly, and ending the day with cooked starches works well because it has all night to digest. But if you eat a cooked meal and then try to have fruit after it, the cooked food will still be slowly digesting when the fast-digesting fruit hits your stomach. This will block the fruit from being digested optimally and can lead to fermentation and overall poor digestion. Many will end up bloated or with stomach aches if they eat fruit after cooked food, so I recommend that once you've switched to cooked food, stick to cooked food for the rest of the day.

If you're still hungry after dinner, eat more cooked starches instead of going back to fruit. The next day, make sure to increase the amount of fruit you eat during the day so you don't face that problem again. It takes time to build up new habits and routines, but keep trying and eventually you'll get the swing of things.

## How much water do I need to drink?

The main thing here is to stay hydrated and happy; that's the goal. So, it's not just about drinking a specific volume of water; it's about making sure you remain hydrated throughout the day and night. Someone living in the desert, for instance, is obviously going to need to drink a lot more water than someone living in a humid rainforest: dry climate verses humid climate makes a big difference. And there are many other factors that come in to play. Most fruits you eat or drink, especially citrus fruits and melons, will help hydrate you, and you can include the water used in smoothies when considering how much you need to drink in your specific environment. But you'll need to drink straight water throughout the day as well, if you want to be properly hydrated.

I recommend drinking water at certain times of the day: when you wake up, about 30mins before big meals, during and after exercise. But the amount needed to remain hydrated will vary for person to person depending on many factors. That's why the best most accurate way to determine if you're drinking enough is to pay attention to the colour and frequency of your urine. You want to be peeing 8-12 times per day on average and you want your urine to be as clear as possible. That's the best measurement. If your urine is yellow, it means "girl you gotta drink up" because you're already dehydrated. If your urine is clear each time, you're doing fine. Drinking water also helps with digestion, so it's good to drink water about half an hour before meals. That'll get your digestive system kicking.

## Do I HAVE to exercise??

The rule is: get out there and move your body! In fitness, consistency is far more important than intensity. What I recommend is to make sure you get outside and get some activity in every day, just move your body for a half-hour or so (could be just playing with your kids, running around the block, cycling, or getting involved in a recreational sport). Then, two or three days each week add some intensity: go for a big ride or a run or a hike and push yourself; or do a home or gym workout and really get the sweat moving.

It's also important not to over-exercise. I see a lot of people who make big health goals, but they push themselves so hard that they eventually burn out and hit the wall. People say to me: "Oh, you must be doing a marathon a day to stay that fit. That's why you're so slim," but, I've actually never done a marathon! I don't exercise nearly as much as most people seem to think I do.

I used to exercise like that, usually twice a day, pushing myself until I could barely move. I'd be icing down my shins at night, always exhausted and in pain. These days, my training is mostly cycling, about 4 times per week, for about 30 minutes or an hour each time, and most of that is only moderate intensity; I'm not always pushing it hard. I'll usually add in a couple of running sessions each week, about 15-30 minutes each at medium intensity, with maybe 5 minutes each time at higher intensity. Every so often, I'll do a running race, usually a 5k, where I'll really push it, but it's generally only every few weeks or once a month that I run a race. So my training isn't huge: I spend more time eating than exercising. :) But I do get out and move every day: going for a walk or a relaxing ride. Overall, I'd say I do about 2 hours of real exercise per week. I also spend, on average, about 8-9 hours per day on the computer. What this means is that if I can be fit and lean on this lifestyle, so can you!

The main idea is that I'm not exercising myself to death. Unless you're aiming for the Olympics, it's not necessary to push yourself so hard. The key to fitness isn't to trash yourself every day with high intensity workouts; it's consistency. Day in and day out move your body, stay active, go outside and play each day, have fun with it and make it something you can sustain for life. If you do that over the long-term, you'll be fit and lean without feeling like you've had to become a supreme-world-athlete to do it.

On RT4, you can let the diet mostly take care of your weight. Eat to stay slim. Exercise for health, fitness and joy. Over the long-term, your body will end up lean from the diet alone; you don't need to exercise in order to lose weight. That's important to understand. Most people exercise because they think that's what they need to do to lose weight, but then they keep eating fatty, unhealthy diets, which is what is really making it hard to stay lean. On RT4, the main focus of exercise isn't for weight-loss: it's for overall health, fitness and stamina.

So when people ask me how I stay slim long term, my answer is: diet. I'd say about 80% of staying slim is diet, and once you're eating right, it's effortless.

**Remember:** you're not going to get fit in two weeks. It takes time. All the fit people you admire and are inspired by have been doing it for years, consistently. So don't get discouraged when you don't see immediate results. Aim for long-term health, stay consistent with a sustainable exercise routine and you'll end up fit and lean for life.

# NETFLIX AND CHILL

Make sure to get lots of rest, relaxation and good sleep. Your body needs down time. After a workout, or activity of any kind, it's important to let our bodies rest and return to homeostasis. Exercise and rest must be balanced, but this doesn't mean equal amounts of time for each the amount of time you spend at rest should be much more than the amount of time you spend exercising.

If you observe animals in nature, they spend the vast majority of their time at rest, which allows them to have the energy they need when they need it. It's also important to notice that animals in nature, even though they spend so much time laying around, aren't overweight for their species (this reinforces the truth that weight-balance and maintenance comes from diet, not exercise).

These days a lot of people sleep as little as possible, but if you look closely you'll notice that most of them are getting through the day hyped up on stimulants like caffeine. Their bodies are begging them for rest, but they're not listening, so they keep pushing and pushing themselves until they get sick enough that they're forced to get some bed rest. When we continuously don't get enough sleep, we really do pay for it: we become drowsy, irritable, we lose concentration, we become less productive in everything we do, and we also set ourselves up for weight gain. Most people are so chronically tired, they've forgotten what it's like to have real, bubbling energy, or to have a sharp and focused mind. They go through their days half-awake, so they're only really half-living.

It's also not just the amount of time spent sleeping and resting that's important; it's about the quality. Exercising a little each day helps you sleep soundly and so does eating enough calories during the day. If you're not doing either of these, you'll probably find it more difficult to get to sleep at night, and you probably won't sleep as well when you do.

Lack of rest and sleep have a big impact on our nervous system. Learning to rest your body and your mind is very important for mental health. Without enough rest, our neurons can become depleted in energy and our brains can end up loaded with the toxic byproducts of cellular activities. Modern scientists have shown that there are pathways in the brain that function much like the lymphatic system to clear out waste from the brain's metabolic activities. Just as lymph fluid carries waste out of our bodies, cerebrospinal fluid carries waste from your brain. Scientists have also shown that sleep is what allows the cleaning process to take place. Lack of sleep leads to cognitive problems, mental challenges and many psychological disorders; and it might also be one of the causes for some of the most serious neurological diseases, like dementia and Alzheimer's disease.

Why else might we want to make sure we're getting enough sleep? Lack of sleep tends to inhibit the production and regulation of human growth hormone (GH), which is responsible for stimulating cell reproduction and regeneration (it's instrumental in skin-renewal, for instance). GH is like nature's little beauty-injection! And it's shown that the largest GH secretions occur during sleep. So make sure to get your beauty-sleep, literally!

Ok, so it's obviously important for our health to get enough daily sleep, but how much do we need? I recommend around 8-10 hours per night, every night. But that doesn't mean going to bed at midnight and waking up at 10am. Going to bed early and waking early is very good for your health. Our immune system functions optimally if we get to sleep by 10pm (at the latest!). Most physical repair takes place between approx. 10pm and 2am, and then from 2am to 6am we enter a stage of psychic regeneration. Lack of sleep, and disordered sleeping will weaken your immune system and increase your chances of disease. So get your sleep girls! :)

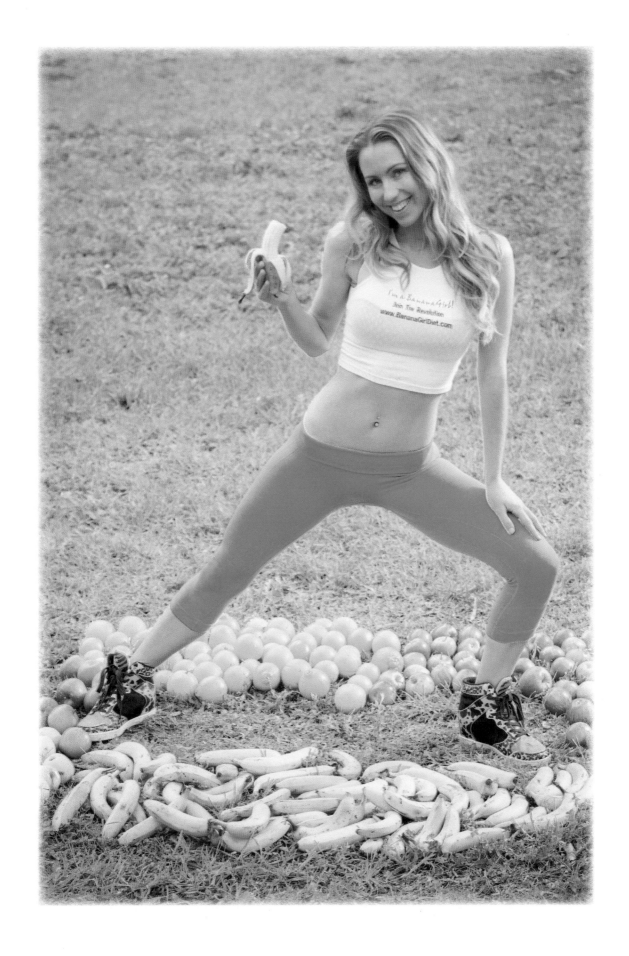

# SUNSHINE

Make sure to get outside, breathe in the fresh air and take in some sun. This will help get you all the vitamin D you need, and it'll improve your skin and your mood! Vitamin D is a very important vitamin, and like B12 deficiency, it's an epidemic in many places, especially northern countries. For instance, one recent study showed that 42% of American adults are vitamin D deficient.

One of vitamin D's major roles is that it helps to promote strong bones, because it increases the amount of calcium absorbed in the gastrointestinal tract and stimulates osteoblastic activity (osteoblasts are cells that synthesise bone). So getting enough D, along with calcium from plants (not from milk) is the best way we can combat weak bones or osteoporosis. Vitamin D also protects against some pretty severe diseases, including several kinds of cancer, heart-disease, diabetes and autoimmune diseases.

Vitamin D is actually not an essential dietary vitamin, because it's synthesised by the body when we get exposure to sun. The sun acts on the skin and our body converts cholesterol (not dietary cholesterol, but the natural cholesterol produced in your body) into vitamin D. This means that the natural way to get vitamin D is not through diet, but simply by being outside and getting some sun.

How much vitamin D do you need? A blood level of around 30 mg/ml is ideal for optimal health. If you get tested for vitamin D, most will tell you that you've failed if you're below 30, but the scientific research on vitamin D actually gives us a minimum of around 20mg/ml before our body begins to react to low levels. When our body recognises that we don't have enough active D in our system (once the level drops below 20), it releases a hormone called PTH in order to boost our levels, and this is how standard minimums for vitamin D are calculated: we know we don't have enough when the body is releasing PTH. Like some other vitamins, there's also a danger of getting too much vitamin D, and it's even possible to get vitamin D toxicity if one is supplementing with pills instead of allowing our bodies to synthesise it internally.

It doesn't actually take a lot of sun to get the amount of vitamin D we need, either. 15-30 minutes of midday sun (with a fair amount of skin exposed) should be enough for most people, though there are many factors to consider, like location, sun intensity, skin colour, etc.. In terms of D synthesis, there's no maximum limit to sun exposure: the body will synthesise what it needs and store the rest.

The ability to store D internally means that if you live in certain cold climates, you may be able to get enough sun through the summer months (under ideal conditions) to store enough vitamin D for several winter months. In other places this may not be possible. We're designed to live in the tropics, so when we settle so far from our usual habitat, one of the drawbacks is that we don't get the sun we need. I don't recommend taking vitamin D pills. Not only would it just be another pill to become dependent on, the latest scientific studies are showing that supplementing D may not even be reliable even among patients given high dosages of vitamin D their blood levels won't necessarily rise as predicted. Also, most D3 supplements come from sheep's wool, which makes it not at all vegan-friendly. There are some vegan D3 versions available, but whether they work or not doesn't seem to be fully settled yet.

**Other options:** One option that might be available for some people is to go visit the tropics in the middle of winter for a couple of weeks. Your body stores vitamin D well, so if you can break up the winter months with some relaxation and sunbathing, that might be all you need. Pretty good excuse for a vacation, isn't it!? :)

Another option is to use a tanning bed. But not just any old tanning bed: you'll need to verify that the tanning bed emits the kind of UV light that helps stimulate vitamin D synthesis. Most tanning beds only emit UVA rays, which aren't very effective at encouraging vitamin D synthesis, but certain kinds of beds are set up to emit UVB rays, which do encourage D synthesis. If you can find the right kind of tanning bed, this seems to be a very good option during long winters.

*"Men and women in bathing suits who were exposed to a 1-MED dose of UVB radiation exhibited increases in blood concentrations of vitamin D that were equivalent to those observed with doses of 10 000-20 000 IU of vitamin D. Therefore, 1 MED is equivalent to 10-50 times the recommended adequate intakes, which are 200, 400, and 600 IU for children and adults <50 y, 51-70 y, and ≥71 y of age, respectively. Studies reported that exposure of 20% of the body's surface to either direct sunlight or tanning bed radiation was effective in increasing blood concentrations of vitamin D3 and 25-hydroxyvitamin D3 [25(OH)D3] among both young adults and older adults. Indeed, Chuck et al (33) suggested that the use of UVB*

*lamps in nursing homes in Great Britain was the most effective means of maintaining blood concentrations of 25(OH)D. . . . We found that tanners in Boston had 25(OH)D concentrations (100 nmol/L) that were >150% higher than those of nontanners (40 nmol/L) at the end of the winter."*

It appears, then, that aside from direct sunlight, the best option for vitamin D synthesis is the use of a UVB tanning bed.
**There is one other interesting option:** D2 derived from fungi. It's actually possible to get D2 from eating mushrooms that have either been "sun-soaked" or treated under a UV lamp, and you can even try that at home. It's still uncertain how well this works though, so sunlight or UVB tanning beds are still the best options by far.

Soaking up the sun isn't just about vitamin D though; it's also about getting out and reconnecting with nature, and about enjoying life a little more. Most people these days spent the vast majority of their time indoors, in stale, lifeless environments. Humans are designed to live in the tropics: that's our natural home. It's our garden of eden (or garden of eatin', if you're anything like me!). We're meant to be outside, playing and nude-baking in the sun all day, not hiding in buildings and covered in clothes, getting almost no sun and hardly playing at all. We've become so detached from nature that most of us feel separate from it, but we're not. We're part of nature, so get out there and remind yourselves of that. Take off your shoes and socks and walk barefoot; strip down and get some nude sun baking in. Reconnect. :)

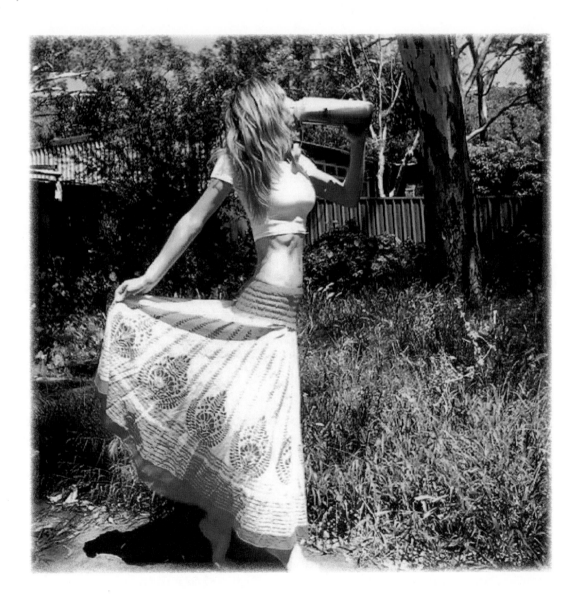

# HOW RT4 WAS BORN

This is where one of my favourite health-inspiration comes in: my mum! She's been there with me all along this health journey, through the lows and the highs. In 2008, she became vegan, and years later she's still a strong ethical vegan. I was doing an all raw lifestyle and thriving, but my mum had only adopted a partly raw lifestyle. Yet she was seeing great results too. She suffered from chronic eczema for years, and when she adopted a high carb vegan lifestyle her eczema vanished. She lost about 12 kilos, her skin improved out of sight, her body looks amazing, and she's healthier every day. It was my mum who one day casually coined the term "Raw Till 4." Once she said that I knew the name was a winner! I spent the next few years structuring and refining the program and today it is a lifestyle that thousands of girls around the world enjoy and thrive on.

This is how Raw Till 4 was born. It comes from years of experience, coaching and observation. It's results-based, and it's something everyone can put into practice. It's not just a good theory: it actually freakin' works!

## YOU'VE BEEN LIED TO...

No one likes to hear that but yep, it's true. You've been lied to most of your life and now it's time to dive deep beneath the surface and reveal the truth. There's a lot of misinformation out there girls mostly because the meat and dairy and diet industries who will tell you anything to get you to buy their products. Most girls believe so many things about diet and lifestyle that just aren't a fact, so let's clear some space in our brains by cleaning out the garbage and taking the stinky scraps to the compost.

## THE CHUBBY TRUTH ABOUT FAD DIETS

Over the years I have had thousands, literally thousands of girls come to me with stories of their fluctuating weight on these anti-life diets. The pushers of these deathly diets show many impressive looking before and after shots of their followers getting leaner and promising you similar results. What they don't explain to you is that their weight loss is temporary hydration/water weight aka dehydration. That's why you will see muscle definition on some of the girls within a month or two because their muscle was already close to the surface. Bodybuilders do this all the time: it's called 'cutting' where they dehydrate themselves before a competition to look ripped on stage.

Sounds great right? You don't need that pesky water making you look fat right?! Wrong. That water is important hydration for your cellular health, it is vital for your health and well being. Any water weight loss that is achieved through calorie restriction is always temporary. What they don't tell you (or show you) is that after under-eating and over-exercising for months you are heading for a massive binge period plus subsequent weight rebound. It is inevitable.

When you don't meet your bodies nutrient requirements by under-eating eventually your survival instinct will rebel to balance that deficit you forced onto your body. When you create weight loss through forced calorie restriction you also create a lazy metabolism and teach your body to hang onto fat reserves or build them back incase of another famine.

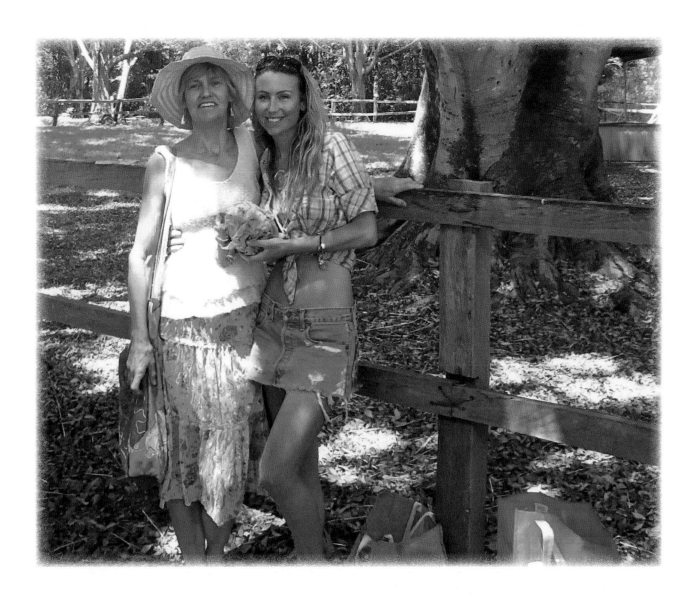

# THE QUICK FIX
# (THE MYTH OF OVERNIGHT HEALTH)

There's no shortcut to becoming your leanest, fittest, healthiest self but the diet industry thrives by keeping that illusion alive. They'll tell you that you can be healthy, with ease, in just 30 days! So-called "health-gurus" tell you that you can become healthy just by coming to their retreat, or by juice-fasting for a week, or by buying their expensive superfood supplements! They tell you that you can lose 50lbs in 30 days, and keep it off, with some magic cure. It's all nonsense.

Think about it this way: It took years, maybe even decades, to get into the unhealthy state you're in. Is it realistic to think that a couple of weeks of eating well or exercising or taking some tonic is all it's going to take to become truly healthy? Of course not. It's going to take time and effort and consistency and knowledge. *Health is a lifestyle. It's not a "fix." That's the first thing we need to understand.*

One of the most common questions I get from newcomers to this lifestyle is: "Why am I not losing weight fast enough!?" The thing is, if we're just coming to this lifestyle now, it means that we haven't been healthy up to this point. If you're like me, you've probably abused your body with calorie-restriction, stimulants, medications or recreational drugs, low-carb diets, and all kinds other things. When I came to this lifestyle, I was totally out of balance, both mentally and physically. Even if you're not in such bad shape as I was in, your body is probably out of balance too.

What goes up, must come down. Every action has its reaction. If we've brought ourselves to a state of dis-ease over years, it's likely going to take years to heal. I know this isn't what most girls want to hear, but I'm not here to lie to you that'll never help you find health, happiness and hotness. I'm here to tell you the cold hard truth.

We need to be consistent, day in and day out, long-term. If you look at the healthiest girls in the world, you'll see right away that they've been working at it for years. Health takes years, and so does fitness (especially fitness!).

But don't let yourself be a victim. You might not become the leanest, healthiest, fittest version of yourself overnight, but if you commit to this lifestyle you will get there, and unlike the popular fad dieters, you'll be able to be healthy for the rest of your life. If you try to cut corners and cheat and only go for the quick-fix empty promises, you'll end up a sucker for the diet industry forever. It's time to give that corrupt diet industry the middle finger by stepping up and becoming truly healthy!

# CALORIE RESTRICTION FOR WEIGHT LOSS?

This is the big one! It's the queen of lies in the diet industry, and it's an issue that's very close to my heart. Before this lifestyle I had been restricting calories most of my life because that's what I thought I needed to do to be healthy and lean, but I didn't even start to be healthy until I finally saw through this fat lie. Now I eat as much as I want, consistently more than I've ever eaten in my life, and yet I'm leaner, fitter and healthier than ever! I've dropped over 40lbs of useless weight. But how can that be if calorie-restriction is the answer to weight loss!?

What actually IS a "calorie"? It's literally a measurement of energy. All it tells you is the potential amount of energy your body might get from a kind of food. It doesn't measure what that food is made of. This is very important, because it helps us understand what calorie-restriction really is it's restricting your body's energy; and not just the energy you need for muscular activity, but also the energy every one of your cells needs to perform its life-giving duties. Without energy, your body cannot function properly. By denying yourself calories, you're cutting off the energy source of all your cells, from the cells that help you digest and assimilate food, to the cells that help your muscles work, to the cells that help you think. Having sufficient energy is the most important thing for the life of your body. You need energy. You need calories. Calories are LIFE.

But what kind of calories? Obviously, eating 1000 calories from fat is not the same as eating 1000 calories from carbohydrates. Both measurements have the potential of 1000 calories of energy for you, but your body isn't going to handle the fat the same as it does the carbs; it won't convert the fat into energy the way it easily converts carbs into energy.

Think about it: if you could get the same energy from fat as you can from carbs, wouldn't athletes drink olive oil before a workout? Oil is the densest form of calories available, so why don't they drink oil to get in calories the easiest way? It's because they know that one calorie doesn't equal another. It all depends on the source of the calories. The reason those eating junk foods might feel better when they restrict their calories, is because they're not stuffing themselves with as much toxic, fatty animal products and chemical-filled processed food. Of course they feel better! But when we're eating the right food high carbohydrate fruits, starches and vegetables, there's no reason to restrict, because you're giving your body the fuel it needs to thrive. On Raw Till 4, the more you eat, the more energy you'll have and the fitter, healthier, and happier you will be long term.

All you have to do is look at examples. Take someone who eats 3000 calories per day of fatty, processed foods and animal products; then take someone who eats 3000 calories per day of high carb plant foods. Are they going to look the same? Feel the same? Have the same energy? A Big Mac' has about the same number of calories as three mangoes, but it doesn't require a degree in nutrition to know that eating three mangoes is better for your body than eating a Big Mac'! How is it that I continue to pound in the carbohydrates, averaging over 2500 calories per day, for years, and I'm lean and fit? The main reason is because I'm eating the RIGHT food and I've been doing that since 2007. I'm eating low fat (about 5%-10% of total calories), low protein (again, 5%-10% of total calories), and I'm not eating toxic junk. I'm eating clean, healthy, nutrient-packed carbohydrate foods, and I'm thriving. Instead of denying my natural hunger for fuel (in the form of carbohydrates), I'm honoring it: I'm giving every cell in my body what it needs to kick ass!

Restricting calories might work to drop a few pounds in the short term, but it NEVER works long term, because calorie restriction is just semi-starvation. Does long-term starvation make sense as a sustainable lifestyle choice? Heck no! Any short term calorie deficit you create through semi-starvation you will pay back later with a binge. You know it's true because you've been there before.

The diet industry survives on the calorie-restriction lie. It's their biggest gimmick. Every diet plan out there teaches you to restrict, restrict, restrict your calories. Then when you inevitably binge out and gain back all the weight you have lost they make you feel like it's YOUR fault, YOU are the failure instead of the shitty starvation plan you were on. No you were just frickin' hungry! That's perfectly natural and is nothing to feel guilty about. You need to honour your hunger drive, not deny it! When you eat the RIGHT calories on the Raw Till 4 lifestyle you do not have to restrict them. You get to eat to your bellies content every single time and long term that nourishment WILL help you transform into the happy, healthy lean individual that you always dreamed of being! How liberating is that? Yep, I'm just a little bit excited over here after decades of starvation. The reality is, when you're convinced that you're the failure, then you're sure to come back to the diet, or to some other diet that also includes calorie-restriction, to try again (probably feeling even worse about yourself then you did the first time). But it's not your fault: the diet doesn't work, because calorie-restriction doesn't work. It never will. Give it up. No one can do it long-term. That's the real problem. No diet that includes calorie-restriction is sustainable long term, because starvation is not the road to health.

As you can tell, I'm very passionate about this issue. It's the number one reason girls fail to reach their health and fitness goals. It's the number one reason girls who come to the Raw Till 4 lifestyle don't stick with it: because they just can't accept that you don't need to and MUST NOT calorie-restrict. We need to get past this lie fruit bats. Until we realize that calorie-restriction doesn't work, and until we realize that what kind of food we're eating is far more important than the amount, we'll never lead a Banana Girl revolution!

# "BUT FRUIT MAKES YOU FAT!" (AKA SUGARPHOBIA)

*"But Freelee! If I eat unlimited calories, even from fruit and starches, I'll get fat! So I have to restrict my calories!"*

Well, girls, it just doesn't work that way. No one gets fat from fruit. No one ever has, no one ever will. The truth is: fruit doesn't make you fat. Starches don't make you fat either. Carbohydrates don't make you fat. FAT makes you fat. Eat a high fat diet, and naturally you will put on fat. Eat a toxic diet and you'll store all kinds of extra weight. Eat a low fat vegan diet, high in healthy carbohydrates loaded with vitamins and minerals, and in time you will become lean and stay lean effortlessly.

Every cell in the human body runs on sugar (glucose), and carbohydrates are the optimal fuel-source. Carbs are easily converted into glucose and used by the body, but fats have to go through a complicated process called gluconeogenesis, where a truckload of energy is used (and lots of waste is produced) trying to convert it into glucose. Which one sounds like the best source of energy? It's easy to see that a high-fat diet isn't the way to go, but a high carb diet is.

There's a lot of "sugarphobia" going around right now mostly because of clever marketing and outright lies by the animal and diet industries. Lots of girls are being told to avoid sugars if they want to be healthy, but it's not the sugars that are making them fat and sick: it's the fatty foods and the animal products!

Girls think they can't eat cake or pastries or donuts because of the sugar. No, you shouldn't eat that junk because of the fat and dairy! Most of the foods girls label as "carbohydrate foods" actually get most of their calories from fat, but girls are tricked into thinking they need to reduce their carb intake, when really they haven't been eating high carb anyway; they've been eating high fat, and they need to reduce the fat. This is why it's important to learn what is actually in the foods you eat: using programs like **www.cronometer.com** can help you see if a food is high in fat or high in carbs.

# Aaaaargh! Why am I gaining weight?

Relax. Short term weight gain is quite common, depending on your background. Don't freak out! If you've been under-eating for years, the body adjusts its metabolism to suit those conditions. When you start eating enough clean, healthy calories and nutrients your body reacts from a state of poor metabolism, and that reaction is to store fat and fluid for future need. If you've been calorie restricting or just not supplying your body with enough nutrients consistently, then your body will be accustomed to that, and will anticipate the same for the future. So what happens is that the body hangs on to everything it can (in the form of fat stores) while maintaining the same poor/slow metabolism. You've temporarily trained your body to be a fat-storer instead of a fat-burner. Your body is trained to anticipate a lack of nutrition, so even when it begins to be given enough calories and nutrients it will still remain in that state for a while (this can vary depending on many factors, in direct proportion to the severity of the past lack of nutrition—could be 6-10 months, could be 2-3 years in some cases like it was for me). After a while on this abundant lifestyle your body will begin to speed up its metabolism, as it heals internally. It needs to become accustomed to receiving adequate calories and nutrition before it will trust you enough not to feel the need to store fat. It takes time for your metabolism to change (the body always works slowly and steadily), but eventually you'll go from a fat-storer to a fat-burner. At that point your body will utilize the fuel you give it fully (utilizing glycogen stores, and not needing fat stores).

This is essentially the core reason why short term weight gain may occur on this lifestyle, and why after a period of time the weight will begin to drop. There are also other weight gains that can happen that have nothing to do with fat: hydration gains, bone density gains, muscle mass gains, increased glycogen stores, more volume of food in your digestive system, water retention, etc. Some girls have been so used to being seriously dehydrated their whole life, when they finally start hydrating their body again, they mistake the increased hydration for fat. And too many girls—way too many girls—are still using that ridiculous and pointless device called a scale! The scale only tells you your weight; it doesn't tell you what that weight is! Too many girls weigh themselves on the scale every day and freak out over every kilo. That's not helpful! Ladies throw out your scale and focus on health instead of trying to micromanage your weight. Stop being so darn superficial and focus on health and long-term your weight will take care of itself. There are NO long term RT4ers who are overweight. That says it all right there. Stick with the program, and even if you gain in the beginning while your body heals, know that you won't be overweight long term. RT4 will naturally burn off your fat without you having to force it to happen through insane exercise. Just embrace the principles of the lifestyle and have patience.

**You are NOT fat. You HAVE fat. Fat is not your name. It is not your identity. It is not who you are. Having fat is a temporary state which you can change at any time.**

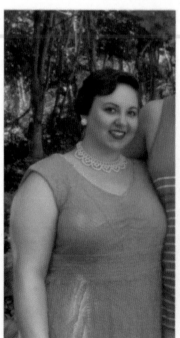
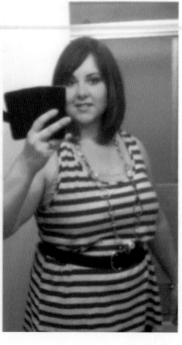
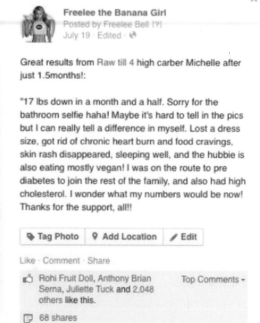

Freelee the Banana Girl
Posted by Freelee Bell [?]
July 19 · Edited · ✥

Great results from Raw till 4 high carber Michelle after just 1.5months!:

"17 lbs down in a month and a half. Sorry for the bathroom selfie haha! Maybe it's hard to tell in the pics but I can really tell a difference in myself. Lost a dress size, got rid of chronic heart burn and food cravings, skin rash disappeared, sleeping well, and the hubbie is also eating mostly vegan! I was on the route to pre diabetes to join the rest of the family, and also had high cholesterol. I wonder what my numbers would be now! Thanks for the support, all!!

🏷 Tag Photo    📍 Add Location    ✏ Edit

Like · Comment · Share

👍 Rohi Fruit Doll, Anthony Brian        Top Comments ▾
Serna, Juliette Tuck and 2,048
others like this.

🗒 68 shares

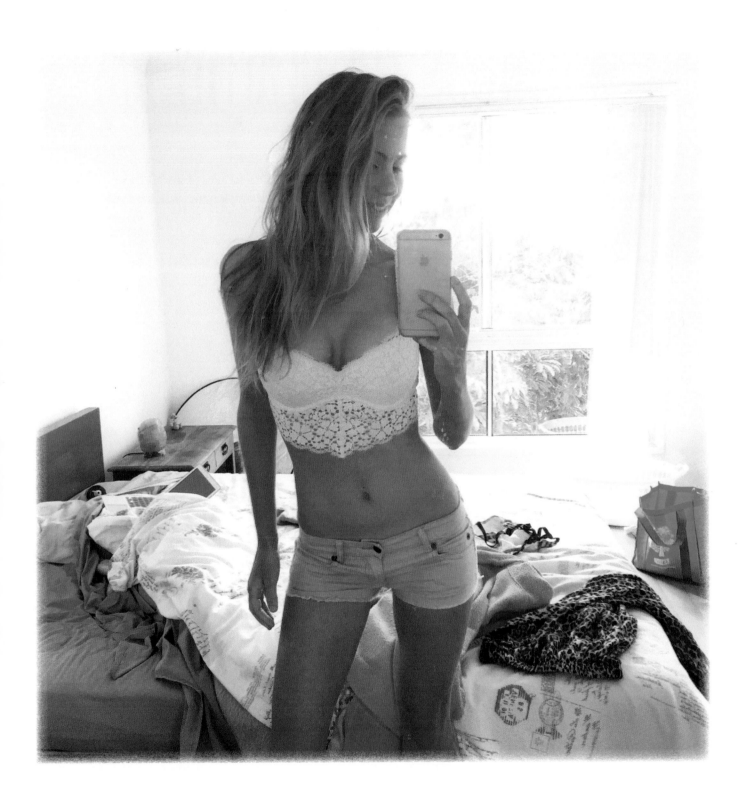

# WEIGHT LOSS THE HEALTHY WAY

*I know many of you are coming to this lifestyle with the desire to lose weight. A big part of my own reasons for adopting this lifestyle was because of my fluctuating weight. I wanted off the roller-coaster ride, and I did manage to get off it.*

*Raw Till 4 is much more than a weight-loss plan: it's a lifestyle, so whether you're underweight and needing to put on some pounds, overweight and needing to lose, or just wanting to get healthier and fitter, long term RT4 will work for you. When we're truly healthy, our bodies will look and feel truly healthy. But since weight loss is such a big motivator for so many people, I want to talk about it specifically here.*

## THROW OUT THE SCALES

Let's talk about the scales, and why they're so inaccurate when it comes to measuring actual fat loss. The problem with scales is that they only measure weight, without telling us anything about what kind of weight they're measuring. When most of us step on a scale and see that the number has gone up since the day before, we automatically think it means that we've gained fat, but it's not that simple. There are many factors that might increase that number on the scale without any extra fat on your body at all. For example:

1. **Hydration.** Being hydrated is always going to increase your weight. Most people in our society are chronically dehydrated (which is why their urine is yellow, when it should be clear). So when people come to this lifestyle and start pounding back the sweet, juicy fruits and finally drinking the water their bodies so desperately need, they will certainly put on a few pounds. It's like your cells going from raisins back to grapes! And that's a good thing. Over half of your total body weight is water, so its vitally important that we stay hydrated. If we go from dehydrated to hydrated, we'll gain weight on the scale, but that's not fat gain!

2. **Food in your system.** This is one of the biggest factors for weight fluctuation that has nothing to do with fat storage. The amount of food in your system can vary significantly from one hour to the next. Your stomach capacity could be anywhere between 1-2 liters, your small intestine is about 7m (22ft) long and your large intestine (colon) is about 1.5m (5-6ft) long and all of them can be more or less full of digesting food at any time. The average person might have between 5-10lbs of food in them at any given time. But the scale doesn't take that into account.

3. **Non-fat substances** being stored in your body, like water-retention.

4. **Glycogen stores** can impact your overall weight, though not as significantly as these other factors.

5. **Muscle mass** is heavier than fat, so people with the same body size but higher percentage of muscle will weigh more than those with more fat. As you get more fit and toned, you might be losing weight from fat, but you'll also be gaining some weight in muscle.

6. **Bone density.** Denser bone weighs more than bone that has been ravaged by osteoporosis-causing animal products. Since the standard western diet promotes reduced bone density, as your body heals the density and weight of your bones will increase.

So when you step on the scale, it's important to realize that it's only giving you a total weight; it's not telling you what that weight is. Is it fat? Water? Food? Muscle? Bone? BMI isn't an accurate measurement of fat either, as it doesn't distinguish between fat and muscle (body builders can even register as obese!).

The pinch test can give some idea of where you're at, and the most accurate method by far is to get a complete DXA (dexa) scan. But you'd be better not to focus on the weight numbers game at all. RT4 is about achieving overall, long-term health. Let the numbers do what they'll do; don't worry about them. Too many people let a little number control their lives. I say: let's have freedom! Throw out the scales! You don't need them. A number doesn't define you (especially such inaccurate numbers), and it does nothing to help you become the healthiest version of yourself.

# THE KEY FACTORS OF WEIGHT LOSS

As we've been discussing, healthy weight-loss is never about starving yourself. Sure it's easy to drop a few kilos by starving your body, but there is always a reaction to every action and your health will inevitably suffer if you try to take shortcuts to weight loss. There's nothing complicated about losing weight the healthy way: it's very simple. So let's talk about what weight loss means.

Did you know that when you lose weight you're not actually reducing the number of fat cells (adipocytes) in your body? Yep, that's right, I still have basically the same number of fat cells in me as I did when I was 20 kilos heavier. What I've lost is all the sludge (fat, toxins and poisons) that was filling up my fat cells. That's important to understand: when you lose fat, you're not getting rid of part of yourself, all you're doing is cleaning yourself out.

Think of it this way: your fat cells aren't fat themselves, they're more like containers for fat. Imagine your fat cells to be like balloons: if you're obese, the cells are full of fatty deposits, water and toxins; if you're lean, those same cells aren't swelled-up with that sludge. That's the difference. When you fill up a balloon, the balloon doesn't change, and when you empty it, it's still the same balloon. So, you are already lean, naturally. You're just hanging on to stuff from the past, literally.

Another important thing is that your fat cells are being renewed constantly the total number of fat cells stays the same, but about 10% of the cells are replaced each year. There is also a "flow" of lipids (fatty molecules; mostly triglycerides) in and out of your adipose tissue (body fat). Fat loss is simply a matter of allowing and promoting the flow out while decreasing the flow in you want less fat and toxins to be directed into storage and you want the current fat and toxins to be cleaned out of your body. That's really all there is to it. If your body is able to get rid of fat and toxins at will, and if you're not adding more through unhealthy dietary choices, you'll lose body fat naturally and easily over time.

The last big thing to realize is that your fat cells aren't your enemy: actually they've been saving your life for years! Yep, that's right, if you're over-weight, like I was, it means that your body has been protecting you from yourself. If you've been abusing and poisoning your body with an unhealthy diet and lifestyle, the only reason you're alive and doing as well as you are is because of your body's amazing ability to store fat and dilute toxins. Your body truly is your best friend, and body fat is just part of its protection system. When you become healthy, your body won't need to be protecting you that way anymore it'll have no reason to store fat or dilute toxins.

I know it's not always easy to hear and think about this kind of stuff, and I know it might make you feel ashamed or down about yourself and your past choices, but the first step forward is to be willing to face the truth, even when it's hard to do. Our lives are in our hands, and we need to be real with ourselves if we're going to start on the path towards true health. That doesn't mean we need to beat ourselves up being hard on yourself is never the way towards health it just means taking ownership of your life and choices and becoming more and more responsible for them. Taking that kind of responsibility is actually very freeing, because it means that nobody else is in control of your life; a scale isn't in control of you; food is not in control of you, you are in control and you have the power to change your life for the better simply by making good choices.

If you're overweight or obese (or on the other side, if you're anorexic or bulimic) it doesn't make you a bad person; it doesn't make you unworthy. It just means you haven't been living up to your true potential... yet. And if you have extra body fat, it just means that your body has been helping you stay alive and healthy enough to get you to this point where you're ready to embrace a truly healthy lifestyle.

Your body is your friend; it loves you. All that's left is for you to begin to love it. When you love your body, you won't want to give it unhealthy foods, or abuse it with stimulants, drugs, alcohol, or in any other way. RT4 is about developing a beautiful and interdependent relationship with your body. It's about respecting yourself and giving your body what it needs to thrive. If you do that, your body will take care of the rest.

I hope this can help you to look at weight loss in a different way: it's not about getting rid of some part of yourself, or about fighting against yourself; it's about giving something to yourself healthy, life giving foods, developing life affirming habits and then allowing your body to do a little of its own house-cleaning.

The way to do this is simple: I see so many people trying to calorie-restrict, or trying to exercise like Olympic athletes every day, or doing all kinds of unhealthy fasts and cleanses, but none of that is needed.

## The factors in weight loss are very basic:
1. You need your lymphatic system to be working.
2. You need cells to be able to transport substances out of your adipose tissue (body fat) so that they can be excreted by the body (in sweat and as waste) or broken down and converted into usable substances; and for that to happen you need energy for your cells (glucose), and vitamins and minerals to allow proper cellular activities.
3. Your cells need to be renewed/replenished regularly in order to continue performing those tasks.

The other main factors are: **consistency and time.** That's the equation for healthy weight loss.

# SHORT TERM VS. LONG TERM

Always think long-term. We want to be healthy and fit and happy for the rest of our lives, not just for the next few months or weeks. Health weight loss takes time, sometimes quite a long time. If you've been abusing your body for years, or even decades (like most of us), it's going to take more than a few weeks to turn that around. Sure, you can aim for short term results, starve yourself and workout three times a day as if your life depended on it, but is that really what you want your life to look like?

When you picture your ideal future self, what do you see? Do you see someone nearly dying every day on the treadmill? Do you see someone deathly afraid of eating too much, denying their hunger all day every day? Of course not. You want what I want: a happy, content, exciting life of abundance! If you follow the usual restriction based diet plans, that ideal life will never arrive. Dieting is simply incompatible with a long-term happy life. The only thing that is compatible is to find a way of life a lifestyle, not a diet that allows you to be consistently healthy, happy, energetic and positive about life.

When I first came to this lifestyle, I wanted instant results, just like everyone does. I wanted to look good and feel good right away! But I realized that I wasn't being realistic. I had to shift my focus and accept that I had treated my body terribly for years and that it would take years for it to recover. Once I shifted my focus and started thinking about long-term health, instead of falling for the magic short term gimmicks, my body started to actually recover and it did take years.

I started this lifestyle in 2007, but I still had lots of learning to do and lots of healing to let happen. It wasn't until a few years later that I really seem to have fully healed. It took time, and I had to be patient and consistent with the lifestyle, but it paid off, and it will for you too.

Now I have a lifestyle I can live for the rest of my life. I can't even imagine wanting to live any other kind of lifestyle. My life is full of abundance, full of health and vitality and energy, and joy. It's also full of play and nature and beautiful friendships, not to mention purpose and drive. All this began by changing my diet: once I was carbed up consistently, everything else started falling into place.

I know that's exactly what you want, and I know you can have it. It will take time, and you'll face challenges along the way, but if you stay carbed up you'll make it!

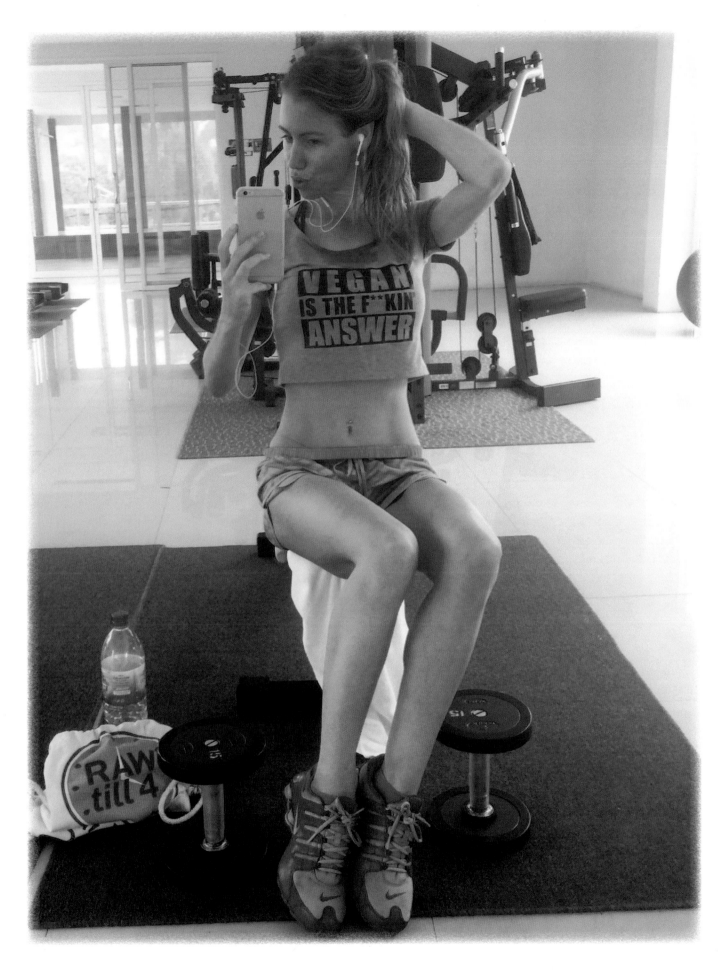

# COMMON EARLY CHALLENGES

*The most important thing to keep in mind here, is that when you're facing a specific issue during your early days/weeks/months on this lifestyle, it is very difficult for anyone to truly know what the cause is without knowing a lot about your health situation and past. This is where keeping a RT4 diary is key! Without a diary it's all about guestimations and it's really not helpful for you or others to be guessing about your food intake or what the causes of your issues are. Objective data is what is really needed in order to address specific health issues, detox symptoms, or other common side-effects of the healing process. So before asking many of these kinds of questions, be sure to start a diary and be consistent with it for at least 2 weeks. When asking for help the most important thing is to be honest! Be transparent and honest and put yourself out there.*

## BLOATING

There can be several reasons why you might be experiencing some bloating in the beginning of this lifestyle. Bad food combining is the most common reason. This can be from eating fruit after cooked food, or from mixing certain kinds of fruit with others, like sweet fruits with fatty fruit or nuts and seeds, or acid fruits with sweet fruits, or melons with anything else (melons should always be eaten alone). Have a look at a food-combining chart for a guide to proper food combining for fruit and veggies.

Another common reason is simply due to our past dietary habits. If you've spent most of your life eating animal products and other high fat processed junk food, then there's probably quite a bit of gunk in your digestive system that needs to be cleaned out. When you start eating lots of fruit and veggies (which have loads of fiber), the cleaning process will start, but it can take time. Until your intestinal tract is cleaned out, the fast-digesting fruit and veggies may be impeded from moving through you as quickly as they should. These can build up and produce gases and can lead to bloating. For those who experience this, it is temporary: once your system is cleaned out your digestion will begin to kick into gear.

Some girls (in our society, most girls) may also have done damage to their gut flora (all the little microorganisms that live in your digestive tracts), and until the body is able to re-balance and repopulate those species, your digestion may not be optimal. Some foods may not digest well, and may lead to buildups of gas. It can take some time for this to heal/re-balance in noobs, especially those who come from more severe ill-health, eating disorders, etc., but everyone who sticks to the lifestyle will experience improved digestion—in time you'll be running like a happy little carb-loaded fruit bat!

Girls should also be careful to pay attention to their menstrual cycle, and not mistake those symptoms for purely dietary symptoms. Bloating and tummy discomfort isn't always due to the food we're eating.

**More reasons for bloating:** youtube.com/watch?v=ZpTRzJzcOLg
**Here is a video on proper food combining:** youtu.be/cgChn26zVaY

## How long will it take to (insert health goal here)?

This question, in all its varieties, is the most common one I get from newcomers to the lifestyle. And I understand; everyone wants to see the light at the end of the tunnel! But it's an impossible question to answer. How long it will take your body to heal can depend on hundreds of factors: it depends on all the details of your past, all your old habits of eating, exercise, stress, sleep, etc., etc.; it depends on everything you're doing now, how closely you're following the RT4 principles, what your life situation is like, etc. The same issue can heal in weeks for one person but take months for another. I see amazing health transformations on this lifestyle all the time. Girls lose weight, clear up their skin, heal their menstrual cycle; girls even reverse type-2 diabetes, chron's, PCOS, IBS, Hypothyroid, etc., etc., but how long it will take is just not something anyone can answer. All anyone can say is: yes, this lifestyle will help you improve your health in a thousand ways, but it will take time.

## Why am I getting acne and/or other detox/healing symptoms?

Acne is a very common healing symptom. Your skin is the largest organ in your body, and when your body is cleaning itself from the inside out, your skin can really show the process to the world. But it is temporary. Long term, your skin WILL clear up, once your body is done its healing and everything is rebalanced internally (including your hormones). Remember, the healing symptoms aren't a reflection that there's something wrong with the principles of RT4; it's a reflection of our past habits. Or even our current food combining or lack of sweating through exercise. Your body will go through some healing when you come to this lifestyle. For some girls that healing is intense and the "detoxing" can be tough. For other girls it'll be only minor. It all depends on where you're coming from and how well you're able to incorporate the lifestyle principles into your life-situation.

## Why do I get dizzy, have headaches, etc. after eating fruit?

This is another issue that may have several causes, but there are some very common ones. The most common reason for dizziness or headaches immediately after eating a large fruit meal is if one still has lots of fat in their bloodstream from their past high-fat diet. The fat coats the receptors of carrier cells, which block insulin from being able to do its job. This inhibits sugar from being transported through the blood to where it's needed, and can lead to a temporary blood-sugar spike. It's not the fault of the fruit, but the fault of the fat from our past dietary habits.

Fluctuating blood sugar levels have been positively linked to migraines, and migraines are found in higher percentages among diabetics than non-diabetics (which demonstrates the link to blood-sugar and insulin). When the blood sugar spikes, the body will react by releasing more insulin, and this can cause a blood sugar spike to be followed by a blood sugar low. The low can then lead to constricting of blood vessels in the brain, and so a headache or migraine will set in. Other triggers can be set in motion by the rebound to a low, including increased blood flow to the brain (the body's attempt to bring more sugar there: more blood = more sugar) which can lead to increased blood pressure and changes in the diameters of the blood vessels in the brain. All of this is due to fat in the bloodstream, a strong reason for adopting a permanently low fat diet! For girls in this situation, what is required is a period of adjustment. You need to allow your body to clean the bloodstream of dietary fat, and this is exactly what RT4 will do—by keeping our intake of fat very low (under 10% of total caloric intake) while also giving our bodies an abundance of nutrients to work with. Another reason for dizziness is simply undereating. Makes sense right? If you're not supplying your body with enough carb calories, your body will start to lack glucose, and a lack of glucose will mean not enough fuel for your brain. When that happens naturally you may feel dizzy or get headaches. The cure is this situation is to carb up! Give your body all the fuel it needs, give your brain all the fuel it needs, and you'll kick ass.

## Why am I craving sweets after dinner?

The simple answer is: you didn't eat enough sweets aka fruit during the day. Cravings for ANY kind of sweet food is your body telling you that it needs more fuel. Every cell in your body runs on glucose/sugar, and if you don't get enough carbs to provide enough glucose to your cells, your body will cry out for more. If you've just eaten a big cooked carb dinner, and your body is suddenly looking for something sweet, it's because it was/is lacking glucose for fuel, and now that it has a big cooked meal to digest, it needs that fuel.

In this situation, it's not good to try to fill the sweet-tooth with fruit, because following cooked foods with raw fruit will almost always cause digestion issues and candida outbreak. The best thing to do is to focus on filling right up with more clean cooked starches that evening (maybe make it a second, small dinner), and then refocus the next day to make sure you get in enough fruit during the day. Cravings at the end of the day mean that we're not supplying our body with all its energy needs, so use those days as motivation to carb up! Really try to get in that minimum of 1500-2000 calories of fruit prior to your cooked meal. It'll make all the difference in the world. When we're truly carbed up and our bodies have all the glucose they need, cravings for sweet things or junk food vanish into thin air, because our body just isn't in need of anything.

## What if I just can't eat that much food?

Oh you will be able to in time. Some girls find it can be difficult in the beginning, because the stomach is accustomed to small-volume foods that provide a lot of calories (mostly in the form of fat). So you need to re-train your stomach to stretch. It's natural for our stomachs to stretch with each meal, and to have a big belly after a big meal. That's normal. It just takes time to get used to it. But also: it's really not that much food, when you think about it. **Here's an example day on RT4:**

**Breakfast:** 8 banana smoothy (850 cals)
**Lunch:** 2 large mangoes and 6 medjool dates (800 cals)
**Dinner:** 2 cups (cooked) of rice with veggies & sauce (550 cals)
**Total calories:** 2200 (Ratio: Carbs 92/Fat 3/Protein 5)

You might be thinking: "8 bananas in one meal! I can't possibly do that!". Ok, then, in the beginning, don't do that. Split it up into two meals of 4 bananas. That should be pretty easy. The best advice is to eat until your full, and then eat a little more.. After a few weeks of doing that, you'll be surprised at how quickly and easily it adapts. After a while you'll be putting back 10 banana smoothies like it ain't no thing!

Now, if you come from a background of severe calorie restriction, and your stomach is the size of a small fist, what can you do? Well, instead of 3 meals in a day, maybe you focus on having 4 smaller meals. Or you can graze: eat about 2 mangoes 6 or 7 times in a day and you'll be at 2100 on just fruit!

Try tricks like these and slowly work your way up to larger meals. But be sure to get in the calories one way or another: your body needs them! Focus on that objective goal of 2100 calories minimum. Success on this lifestyle depends on giving your body enough fuel and enough nutrients, and the only way to do that is to re-train yourself to eat large volumes of high carb foods.

**The Compassionate Vegan**  1 minute ago
I have been a Jenna marbles fan for years, and so I came across your first video about Jenna. when I watched it, I just thought "ugh look at that stupid girl that's just jealous of Jenna. stop showing off your stomach. not everyone can have that" its hard to believe now that I thought that. about a year later, my twin sister went vegan, and I was interested and fascinated. I became vegetarian for a month, then I wanted to make the step to veganism. I needed help, so I remembered your video about Jenna and looked it up and found your channel. then I found other vegan channels. now, 6 months later, I have my own new channel! the celebrity videos I think are the most efficient form if activism. thank you, freelee.

# "JUST LISTEN TO YOUR BODY"

Instead of calorie-restricting (HECK NO), the Raw Till 4 lifestyle recommends unlimited calories from carbohydrates. There is no maximum number of calories per day, but I do recommend an absolute minimum of 2100 calories for girls based on the World Health Organisation recommendations. Anything under that is considered semi-starvation and of course I am not going to endorse that. Some girls who come to the lifestyle don't like the idea of an objective minimum calorie target. Instead, they want to "listen to their bodies" or eat "intuitively." What "listening to your body" really means is "listening to your feelings," and feelings are just body-signals. They let you know when something is working well, or not working well, or when something from your environment is good for you or bad for you. Ideally we should be able to listen to our body-signals and do just fine, but in reality there's a big problem with that: if you're not healthy, and haven't been healthy long-term, your body's signals aren't going to be healthy either! If you're accustomed to calorie-restricting, or to eating fatty foods that are calorie-dense, your body-signals will respond from that state. They're not going to help you become healthier; they're going to help you stay where you are, because that's the state they're accustomed to.

The simplest example of mixed-up body signals are the signals for stomach capacity. Low stomach capacity is common in beginners to the RT4 lifestyle, due to years (or an entire lifetime) of consuming foods that have low volume but high caloric density (like foods with lots of oil or animal products). When switching to a high carb diet, they start eating foods that have high volume but low caloric density (especially fruits and veggies). This means that many girls have trouble consuming enough carb calories in the beginning because their stomach signals are accustomed to such small volumes they get full on very small meals of fruit because they're used to small meals but the calories in the fruit meal might be 1/2 or even 1/4 of the calories in the low volume meals they're used to eating. This leads them to under eat on high carb foods if they just listen to their body.

This is a stage we must work through by increasing the amount our stomach can handle in one sitting so that we can get enough calories from fruit or starches in each meal. Over time it will feel natural and easy to consume 800+ fruit calories in one sitting, because that really is our natural way (our stomachs are designed to expand for that kind of eating), but in the beginning it won't feel natural for everyone.

I also hear girls make statements like: "my body was telling me I needed more fat" or "my body needed animal products." Those kinds of statements are just inexperienced and uneducated. Usually girls are just under-carbed and starving, so their bodies start searching for the quickest, easiest source of high-density calories. When they eat some fatty, junky food, they feel satiated, so they convince themselves that listening to their body was the right answer. But really, all they needed was to eat more calories from fruit or cooked starches and they would've been fine. The term "listening to my body" has become a kind of go-to excuse when girls aren't eating enough of the right foods and take the easy way out. Or they are impatient and want quick weight loss results.

Dr. Douglas Lisle talks about the problems with our body-signals in his book The Pleasure Trap. Your body signals essentially help you do three things: seek pleasure, avoid pain and conserve energy. That's what your feelings are telling you. They're not telling you how to be optimally healthy, lean and fit. It's not your feelings that are going to guide you to health: it's your mind.

Your feelings will direct you to the most calorically-dense stimulating food, for short-term satisfaction. Your feelings want you to get the most instant pleasure, with the least energy spent and the least pain. So in our society, they'll lead you towards super-rich, fatty foods, probably loaded with animal products, because those give you the quickest satisfaction; or if you're vegan, you'll end up going for high fat, "gourmet" vegan foods. In our world it's much easier to go through the drive-in and get a greasy burger than to cook a healthy rice dish for dinner, but going for the easy, greasy food is what I call: "eat now, pay later." Sure, you get immediate satisfaction, but you'll pay in the long run with fat gain, dis-ease and depression.

It's your intelligence that will direct you to the foods that are actually good for you, in the right volume, and it's your intelligence that will help you stay on the lifestyle long term, because you'll know it works, even while you're body is still adapting to it. That's why it's so important to read and learn about health. It's also why I set objective targets for our health.

The other kind of "listening to your body" is generally popular with spiritual girls who mistake lack of energy with calmness and contentment or spiritual-bliss.

In actuality, their mind's are spaced-out from being under-carbed and their bodies have dampened their hunger signals and metabolism so they feel a kind of physical deprivation. They listen to their body and under eat, and this starves their body and mind of energy. They end up thinking of being spacey as a "spiritual" state, but mental clarity and physical energy come from being carbed up, not from starving the body and mind. Eating enough to be physically healthy and setting objective goals based on an understanding of how the human body works isn't non-spiritual or somehow not natural, and being physically fit isn't in opposition to being spiritual. In fact, the most spiritual girls I know are carbed up fruit bats who are full of life and happiness; they're energetic and radiate happiness, compassion and love.

When we're coming from an unhealthy background, and living in the real world, listening to our bodies without objective goals isn't the road to health. We don't just "listen to our car" to know when it needs more fuel or an oil change or new tires; we read gauges that give us objective data. That way we don't need to wait for it to run out of gas before we know to fill it up, or wait for something to seize before changing the oil, or wait for a flat before changing the tires. Why would we just listen to our bodies when we also have objective ways to gauge when we need more fuel, or certain vitamins, or more fiber, or more water, etc.? Hmmm.

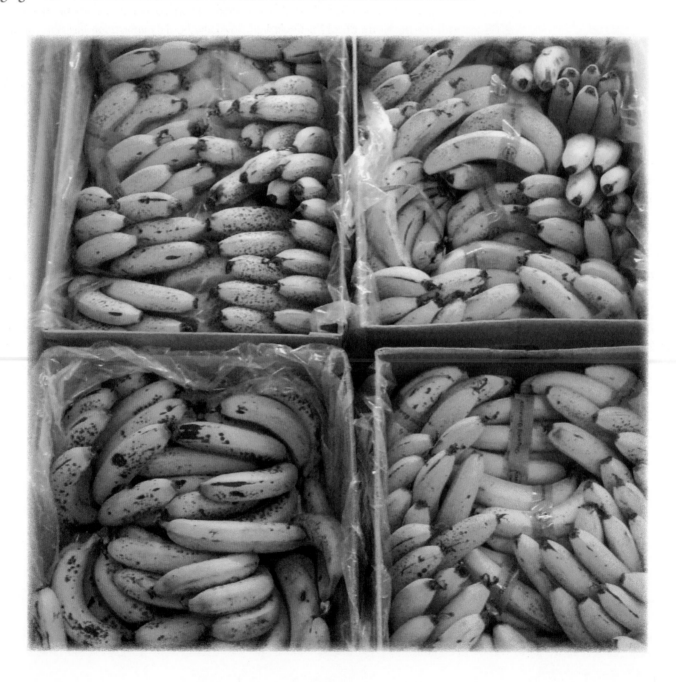

# EMOTIONAL EATING

Emotional eating is something I simply don't subscribe to. I used to think it was legit when I was chronically under-carbed, but now I realize it's rubbish. If you want to eat then you need to eat. The desire to eat is your brain telling you that it's running low on glucose and needs carbs baby! The challenge is eating the right calories in that moment. This is where your mind comes in again. You've got to be discerning. If you get an emotional drive telling you to eat more, then sure, you can go eat fatty pastries or greasy burgers and pizza, or you can stuff your face with chocolate and other junk. But none of that is going to solve the real problem. Every so-called "emotional eater" in the world knows this: binging on junky food never solves the problem. You always want more. But it's not because you're an emotional person, or need a therapy-session: it's because you're not giving your body what it truly needs: carbohydrates! Remember EVERY cell in the human body runs on glucose aka carbs.

Sure there are addictive substances in some of the fatty, greasy foods we can eat, but that's not why we go for them. We go for them because they give us the biggest, quickest calorie hit. But it doesn't matter how big the calorie hit is if its primarily from fat our body and brain will still need glucose from carbohydrates so the emotional drive to eat won't go away and we'll just keep binging (and unfortunately, many will start purging too like I used to).

This is the same reason why girls feel the need for dessert after a big meal. They've filled up on fatty, non-nutritious foods and haven't given their body what it really needs: glucose, sugar. This is why they have a "sweet-tooth." To solve the problem, they give themselves a quick hit of some refined sugar treat, which is usually loaded with fat too! It's an endless cycle, but the answer is simple: emotional eating is rubbish. When you give yourself enough glucose from carbohydrates, the problem solves itself. It's not a desire that needs to be suppressed; it needs to be honored.

So, if you fill up with carbs, does it mean you succumbed to "emotional eating"? No! It just means you did what your body needed, you gave your cells the glucose they needed! When your hunger drive rises up and says: "I need food!", you have to honor that the same way every animal on the planet honors it (they don't go to therapy; they eat their natural food!). You just need to give yourself the right food, the food the human body thrives on.

If instead of this, you punish yourself, and say: "no, you're just being emotional, you need a therapy session," then you start to create a very unhealthy and destructive relationship with your body. You also lower your metabolism. Believe me, I've been there. If you deny what your body truly needs, you'll drive yourself to a very unhealthy place. Be a friend to your body! Be a friend to your brain! Nourish them properly and they'll repay you a thousand times over. Promise.

 **Klairee Berry** 😊 feeling happy
15 hrs · Edited · 🌐

**So the day before yesterday was my 18 Month Veganniversary!!
♡☆♡☆♡☆♡ I would like to thank** Durianrider Durian Rider **and** Freelee the Banana Girl **for making this possible! I have no more candida and IBS symptoms and I have more confidence, clarity and energy than ever before. I have been absolutely loving being able to eat as much as I want everyday while still losing over 13 pounds and counting - and maintaining it. For me to get at and stay at the same weight I would have had to calorie restrict severely and overexercise, but with RT4 I am at peace everyday and workout almost daily because it's fun and feels good.**

# THE LOW CARB CRAZIES

Now that you know a little about protein and fat, it doesn't take much to see why a Low Carb diet is one of the worst things you can do for your health. If you're limiting your carbohydrates, what are you eating? Fat and protein. And mostly fat! Does that really seem like a good idea?

Low carb "gurus" say you'll lose fat by eating fat. Does that make any sense to you? It sure doesn't to me. But, if you wanna get fat, clog your arteries, rev-up cancer cell production and get osteoporosis and diabetes, low carb is for you!

Low carb "gurus" also say that high protein is good for you, and even necessary for your health. It's not. If we don't take in enough carbs and at the same time eat too much protein, the body will go into a state of ketosis. What is ketosis? It's when there is an accumulation of ketones in the blood, which are byproducts of fat oxidation (without enough carbohydrates to convert into energy, the body starts to convert fat from foods and storage, but ketones are the by-product of that kind of metabolism). Ketones are toxic (poisonous), acidic chemicals such as acetone, acetoacetate, and beta-hydroxybutyrate.

Ketosis also results in a loss of appetite; the body basically turns off its hunger signals. It's the exact same state you would go into if you were literally starving to death! This seems to be a kind of protection, so while you die you aren't suffering with such bad hunger pains. And this is the way low carb diets work: they put you into a purposeful state of starvation! Sure doesn't sound like a sustainable diet to me. Ketosis is a very dangerous state to be in as it also increases insulin resistance and glucose intolerance. Insulin resistance is a major risk factor for the development of heart disease, and glucose intolerance has been connected to hypertension and dyslipidemia (an abnormal amount of lipids, like cholesterol or fat, in the blood). When our bodies are in a state of ketosis dehydration will result, due to the kidneys being overtaxed by having to rid the body of excess nitrogen. This can cause dizziness, headaches, confusion, nausea, fatigue, sleep problems, and worsening of kidney problems. I have been in a state of Ketosis myself when I went on a low carb diet years ago my acne increased, I was constantly lethargic, my breath stank, and I felt like crap! I was also having suicidal tendencies.

Whenever you find someone on a low carb diet, you'll also notice that they're depending on stimulants to get through the day. They can't function without their coffee or energy drinks. They're basically wiring themselves up on caffeine, or cordyceps, dimethylamylamine or other stimulants. Some also take fat-burning pills, ECA stacks, clenbuterol, and all kinds of other chemicals in order to trick the body into exerting energy (without actually supplying real energy to the body). The low carb lifestyle just isn't sustainable long-term, so they always end up hitting the wall and crashing. Then the weight piles back on, and they become even sicker than before.

## Five reasons Low Carb Diets make you fat in the long-run.

1. Low carb diets lead to binging and turn the body into a "fat storer." When we starve our brains and bodies of what it needs (glucose) we'll become binge-prone, always. And our metabolism will slow right down, so as soon as we start eating real food again the first priority of the body will be to store everything it can!
2. The fat you eat is the fat you wear. Eating fat to lose fat is rubbish! Total nonsense. It doesn't work. The fat you eat goes right into storage (as body fat, or clogged in the bloodstream, etc.), every time.
3. Low carb kills your drive to exercise. Without carbohydrates your cells are starved of glucose, so your energy is going to drop right along with your metabolism. Stimulants can make you think you have energy for a while, but eventually your body will shut down. Actually, the stimulants will just get you there faster.
4. Low carb diets initially fool you into thinking you're losing fat. People go on a low carb diet and immediately drop a few pounds, maybe even a few kilos. But what they're actually losing initially is water-weight from dehydration. This instant-gratification tricks them into thinking the diet works, when in reality they're just experiencing the initial stages of starvation.
5. Your body cannot efficiently, safely or sustainable burn fat in the absence of carbohydrates. We need a steady supply of carbohydrates in order to burn fat efficiently. Without the carbs, all we're doing is starving ourselves. Sure, you might lose fat, but you'll pay for it later (and as soon as you crash and are forced to stop the low carb diet, it'll all come back anyway).

## If you're still not convinced, here's a few sources to read-up more on the dangers of low carb diets:

- Dr. Joel Fuhrman on Low Carb Diets at www.diseaseproof.com
- The Paleo Diet is Uncivilized (and Unhealthy and Untrue) and "High Protein Diets," by Dr. John McDougall
- Analysis of Health Problems Associated with High-Protein, High-Fat, Carbohydrate-Restricted Diets, by PCRM

## What do I do if my family/partner/friends aren't supportive of this lifestyle? What resources can I share with them?

This is a very common question, and one of the biggest difficulties of the lifestyle. Social disapproval can be a bit shit in the beginning. We all have friends and family and loved ones who we love, and we care about our relationships with them. When we become vegan, and when we start eating differently from them it can sometimes cause them to react negatively towards us. I see many girls struggling with disapproval from their parents, if they're young, or from their partners and friends. There's really only one simple answer though: you've just got to do what you know is right for you! You can't change the way other girls think or feel, or the way they treat you. You've got to follow your own path and find the strength within you to embrace it regardless of what others say. You want to be healthy, and you've finally found the way to do it: don't let others talk you out of it or bully you into conforming to society's unhealthy habits.

For sure dealing with disapproval can be a pain in the beginning, it does get easier with time. As you start really demonstrating the results of this lifestyle, girls might still disagree with you, but it gets pretty darn hard for them to ignore those results. Long term RT4ers are shining examples of true health, from top to bottom, inside and out, so even if people still argue against the lifestyle, they'll have a hard time explaining how it is that you're so vibrant and healthy! So, focus on that, focus on long term health, and ignore the haters or doubters who really are just uneducated.

When it comes to boyfriends, it can be a real challenge. If you got into a relationship before going vegan or embracing RT4, and your boy isn't interested in joining you on that path, it can put real strain on the relationship. Each person has to decide for themselves what to do. For some, the right decision will be to leave the relationship if it becomes unsupportive or divisive. For others, they might find ways to balance the relationship despite the differences that come up. The main thing is to be open and transparent with your boyfriend and keep an open dialogue. If you don't have that, lettuce be honest the relationship is probably doomed anyway. So open up and explain to your partner what you're doing and why you're doing it. Show them videos, read plant-based health books together, watch documentaries together. Help them understand the lifestyle, and why you've chosen it. How they choose to respond is not in your control, but you will have done your best. Cut him loose if he makes excuses and won't come to the party, you ain't got time for that!

For young RT4ers who are still living with their parents and aren't yet free adults, the same idea applies: talk to your parents, share information with them, share videos and documentaries and books with them. They'll probably be worried that you won't get enough nutrients or have other concerns about the lifestyle, so the best thing you can do is first educate yourself, and then help educate them. Show them websites from respected plant-based doctors (McDougall, Esselstyn, Caldwell, Greger, Barnard, etc.), show them long-term successful RT4ers so they can see healthy girls on the lifestyle. Really help them see what you see, and show them the reasons why you've chosen this lifestyle. If you're passionate about veganism, show them documentaries on why veganism is essential; show them Gary Yourofsky's speech; watch Earthlings with them; explain to them the ethics behind veganism and why it's important to you. And, if after all that, your parents still insist that you consume animal products, you have the right to say no. You can refuse to eat your animal friends. No one has the right to force you to participate in something you are morally opposed to. If you continue to run into problems with them, reach out to the RT4 community for advice and assistance and support.

**VeganMangoMcD Tonya** 14 hours ago (edited)
**+Freelee the Banana Girl** Thanks for the mention at 4:40. I am now down from 317 lbs starting April 17, 2014 to as of today, October 11, 2014, 263 lbs. I feel awesome! No more acne, my skin is smoother and healthier. I have crazy amounts of energy all the time and I used to feel like I needed coffee all the time. Before starting this lifestyle I was also undergoing various medical treatments for a pituitary microadenoma- all of the meds either made me too sick or just flat out did not work. Six months on the RT4 lifestyle and the symptoms are gone. I want to get my blood work/hormone panel done to confirm it, but I really think it is gone or it has shrunk so much that it is not a significant factor in my health at this time. I am still running occasionally but have gotten into cycling and weightlifting more. Have you checked out Jehina Malik? She has videos on YouTube. She is a vegan since birth and an IFBB pro bodybuilder. Very inspiring! I can't imagine going back to meat and dairy now!

# COMMON HEALTH CONCERNS

## Do I need to supplement vitamin B12?

Maybe. Maybe not. The first thing to know is that B12 isn't a vegan issue. 40% of the population of the USA are B12 deficient, and less than 1% of the population is currently vegan. So B12 deficiency is a big problem for nearly half of the population (vegan or not). You can get tested to verify if you're B12 deficient (go for the Urinary MMA test, as it's the most accurate). If it turns out you're B12 deficient, you'll definitely need to supplement. If you haven't gotten a blood test, or can't get one for whatever reason, it's safe to supplement B12 anyway, just to be sure, as your body will eliminate any excess B12 in your system.

**There are two types of B12 supplements that are recommended.**
1. A sublingual: a single tablet that goes under the tongue.
2. An intramuscular injection (shot), which generally goes into the upper arm.

Both of these methods bypass the absorption process, and bring the B12 vitamin directly into the bloodstream. The injection is the best option, to guarantee that you're getting all the B12 you need.

There are many symptoms that may come up from lack of B12, two main ones are chronic fatigue and depression. It may be quite often that girls have these symptoms and never make the connection to a B12 deficiency. When you supplement B12 you may just find these symptoms greatly improve, and you may find other positive effect too, like more efficient fat-loss, for instance. I feel B12 supplementation accelerated my fat loss.

## Don't we need healthy fats?

There are a lot of myths involved in the "healthy fats" idea. The truth is, the human body needs very, very little dietary fat. In fact, the less the better!

There are three types of dietary fat: poly unsaturated, mono unsaturated and saturated. Saturated fats are never good for our health. Any intake of saturated fats causes the liver to start pumping out extra "bad cholesterol" (LDL), and saturated fats immediately damage the endothelial lining of the arteries when eaten. Most plant fats are unsaturated, but they can be either mono or poly unsaturated. There is no need for either saturated or monounsaturated fats in our diet. So the only kind of fat we need from diet is polyunsaturated, and there are actually only two fatty acids that we need from diet at all: alpha-linolenic acid (an omega-3 fatty-acid) and linoleic acid (an omega-6 fatty acid). These are known as Essential Fatty Acids (EFA).

We actually need a very tiny amount of either omega 6 or 3. Standard requirement is usually given at 1.1-1.6 grams per day, but actual requirements are probably more around the 0.4-0.5 grams per day. So we're dealing with somewhere around 1-2% of total calories.

The important thing isn't about getting a lot, but just making sure that the ratio of 3 to 6 is as close to 1:1 as possible. The problem with girls on a Standard American Diet is that they get too much omega-6, so their ratio is way off. The solution from mainstream nutritionists is to encourage them to eat more omega-3s to balance the ratio, which is utter nonsense because they're already loaded with fat! The "healthy fats" movement is really nothing but clever PR for the animal industry, designed to get girls to keep buying eggs and fish and other nonsense products, and it has spread into vegan circles for absolutely no reason. The real solution is for girls to cut down on their omega-6s to bring the ration back into balance. This means doing the RT4 diet correctly.

*"The safest and healthiest way to get your EFA [essential fatty acids] is in their natural packages of starches, vegetables, and fruits. Here they are found in the correct amounts in protected environments surrounded by vitamins, minerals, fibers, antioxidants, and other phytochemicals to make them balanced nutrition."*—Dr. John McDougall

Just focus on getting enough calories from carbohydrates—from fruit, starches and veggies—and you'll get all the omegas you need, and most importantly, in the right ratio.

# THE PROTEIN MYTH

Ah, the favorite question of non-vegans: "But where do you get your protein!?" If only I had a dollar for every time I hear that question. Protein, protein, protein. It's a big buzz word. But do girls actually know how much protein the human body needs?

Did you know that the World Health Organization recommends only 0.66 g/kg per day as a protein requirement for healthy adults? For most girls this means somewhere between 30 grams (100lb/45kg person) to 50 grams (175lb/80kg person). This means that the average healthy adult only needs between 120 and 200 calories from protein per day! If the 100lb person is eating 2500 calories per day (remember that the UN defines famine as anything under 2100), then this means only 5% of total calories from protein. If the 175lb person is eating enough to be healthy and fit, they'll need well over 2500 calories per day; likely closer to 4000, which would mean 50 grams of protein is also 5%. And remember, this is an average requirement, not a minimum requirement.

Did you also know that human breast milk only has about 6-7% of its calories as protein? (cow's milk has more than double that, by the way). So when we are babies and we're doubling our weight in 5 or 6 months, the food we're designed to eat (mother's milk) is giving us far less protein than the average adult SAD eater. If we only need 6-7% as growing babies, why would we need more as adults?

## *So now you know how much protein you need (it's not much, is it?!). How much is TOO much protein?*

Dr. T. Colin Campbell's research shows that too much animal protein, specifically casein (which represents about 87% of the protein in dairy) is directly linked to cancer cell production, osteoporosis and other major health issues.

*"My laboratory in a long series of studies conducted over more than two decades showed that the growth of experimental cancer is markedly stimulated by the consumption of animal-based casein, the main protein of cow's milk. This occurs in part because this animal source protein stimulates the production of the same growth hormone that spurs childhood growth. Plant based proteins tend not to promote these events, not at least when fed at levels typically found in the whole foods, plant based diet. . . . Increasing body growth may be useful for . . . growing children faster, but it also means growing cancer cells faster, improving conditions for heart disease and speeding up aging each of which has been documented. One of the primary mechanisms for [the cause of osteoporosis] is that animal protein tends to create an acid-like condition in the body, called 'metabolic-acidosis'. To combat this condition, the body draws upon its most readily available acid buffer, namely calcium in our bones. As the calcium is extracted to neutralize the excess acid, our bones are weakened."*

Dr. Campbell shows that diets containing more than 10% of calories from animal-protein are linked to increased cancer growth, so it's not just that we need a minimum amount of protein; there's also a maximum amount we shouldn't consume more than. But we don't have to struggle to make sure we hit the perfect amount every day: nature has done that for us! Fruits and vegetables average about 5-7% of their calories from protein, potatoes about 6%, rice about 7.5%, corn about 9%, grains like quinoa about 15% and these are all staple Raw Till 4 foods! What is just as important though, is that Dr. Campbell's research shows that plant-proteins don't cause the same cancer growth and other health issues as diets with the same amount of animal-proteins, even at higher levels, so if we adopt a plant-based, vegan diet, we really don't need to worry about how much protein we're getting! The foods we eat on the RT4 lifestyle will give us the kind of protein we need in exactly the right amounts.

## Are plant and animal foods the only place we get protein from?

Well, I don't know about you, but I actually get most of my protein from human flesh! Haha, it's true: most of the protein your body uses is manufactured internally from recycled cells and digestive enzymes. So there's no escaping it: we're all cannibals after all!

Seriously though, most of the proteins the human body uses are created by our bodies from our bodies. This is why only a few of the amino acids the human body uses need to come from dietary sources. These are called "Essential Amino Acids" and typically eight or nine are listed. But even of these, the science isn't conclusive that we need them all from diet, or how much of each one we need. Some girls say that if you're vegan you need to make a special effort to get enough of the right amino acids by eating certain plant-foods in exactly the right amounts and combinations. This is rubbish and debunked time and time again.

*"It was once thought that various plant foods had to be eaten together to get their full protein value, a method known as 'protein combining,' or 'complementing.' We now know that intentional combining is not necessary to obtain all of the essential amino acids."*

The main idea is: we don't need a lot of protein, we especially don't need protein from animal products, and if we eat a plant-based diet, we don't need to make any special effort to get enough protein just eating enough fruits, grains and vegetables is all we need to do.

**Please educate yourself further by checking out the links below:**

https://nutritionstudies.org/protein-juggernaut-deep-roots/
https://nutritionstudies.org/mystique-of-protein-implications/
https://www.drmcdougall.com/misc/2007nl/apr/protein.htm
https://youtu.be/aR9iz8d_Dj4
https://nutritionfacts.org/topics/protein/
https://nutritionfacts.org/topics/animal-protein/
https://nutritionfacts.org/topics/plant-protein/

**Natalie Plamondon**  2 minutes ago (edited)
Hey Freelee! I know you get hundreds of comments a day and you may not see this, but I wanted to thank you with all of my heart. I have been struggling with eating disorders off and on now for eight years. Binging, purging, anorexia, crash dieting, ect. I started following your videos since this past march and my entire life has changed. I fell off the lifestyle a few times, but I kept watching your videos and I kept trying. I'm now following your wisdom to the fullest and may I say I am the fullest. No more cravings, I don't feel bad, I have tons of energy, I run three to four times a week, and I'm not binging or purging. Eating my giant mono meal of bowled potatoes with garlic right now!!!! If I could fly to Australia and give you a hug I would!! My life is forever changed. Thank you so much girl!!! Much LOVE <3 keep posting the good stuff. You get me through my week friend.

## What about calcium, iron, etc? (and: "cronometer says I'm low in ____ nutrient.")

There are so many concerns about individual nutrients in the health world, but most of them are just scare tactics to get you to buy some shitty expensive product. In reality, all we need to do is eat a proper, healthy diet of abundant fruit, starches and veggies to get all that we need. A good book to read on the problem with focusing on individual nutrients instead of on overall health is T. Colin Campbell's book Whole: Rethinking the Science of Nutrition.

I highly recommend using **http://cronometer.com** to track your food intake, especially in the beginning of your journey on this lifestyle, but many girls who start using cronometer (or similar tracking programs) become concerned because the default settings will tell them that they're lacking in a certain vitamin or mineral. In some cases, the default settings are based on flawed or biased science or have been unnecessarily effected by food industry propaganda. The default setting for calcium is a good example of this. It is also impossible to know exactly how much nutrition is in each piece of fruit we buy. The standard amounts shown in cronometer are the nutrition world's best guesstimate or average based on standard testing, but the banana you have might have more or less of any given nutrient than cronometer shows. So the main point is that cronometer is best used to guide us in the big picture: number of calories, macronutrient ratios, and a general sense of vitamins and minerals, but it's going to be less accurate for specific nutrients, specific amino acids, etc. The only truly accurate way to determine if we have vitamin or mineral deficiencies is to get regular blood tests done. But anyway let's address a couple of popular concerns:

# CALCIUM

As far as calcium goes, the dairy industry has been very successful at creating concern over nothing in that area. Here's some good quotes, and studies, and other materials.

**Article by Dr. McDougall explains:** https://www.drmcdougall.com/misc/2007nl/feb/whenfriendsask.htm

**Couple of quotes from an article and a study:**
*"A 1992 review of fracture rates in many different countries showed that populations with the lowest calcium intakes had far fewer fractures than those with much higher intakes."* http://pcrm.org/health/health-topics/preventing-and-reversing-osteoporosis
*"Calcium intake is much lower in Asia and Africa than in the United States and Europe, mainly due to the exceedingly low intake of milk and dairy products. However ... the prevalence of osteoporosis, especially hip fracture, is currently much higher in Western countries than in developing Asian countries"* http://www.ncbi.nlm.nih.gov/pubmed/15775506

The human body really doesn't need anywhere near as much calcium as we're taught it does. The concern over "getting enough calcium" is nothing more than a very successful marketing ploy by the dairy industry (as McDougall explains in the article above). On the RT4 lifestyle we get easily enough calcium just from an abundance of fruit and veggies, and by avoiding animal proteins we avoid the problem of our body leeching calcium from our bones (see "**Forks Over Knives**" for more on that issue).

Krysia Dorothy  4 hours ago
Freelee, you have changed my life! I am only 17 and I have never dealt with any food related health issues, except for bulimia. You helped me completely rid of my bulimic tendencies, and introduced me to the best lifestyle in the world! I am so glad I found you at my young age. Because of you, I know that I will live a long healthy life that is full of compassion for animals, humans, and the planet. Thank you for being the beautiful person that you are! You're changing the world! #eatalldaplants

Read more

Reply · 41 👍 👎

# IRON

It is possible to be iron deficient. But it is also possible to get too much iron. The human body has no way to excrete excess iron, so whatever amount is absorbed stays in us and is either utilized or just builds up. Excess iron in the brain has been linked to neurological diseases like Alzheimers, and extra iron in the body is linked with cancer growth. So if you're concerned about iron, the solution isn't simply to go straight to supplementing. With iron, it is important to get accurate blood tests done to determine if you're deficient. Find out WHY you are losing blood? If you are deficient, there's no real need to supplement, the better option is just to focus on eating an abundance of fruit and veggies. Make sure you are eating enough! Make big green smoothies in the morning, or have green juice as a snack between meals. Remember, don't blame the RT4 lifestyle for making you iron-deficient if you don't have any blood tests from your previous meaty diet for comparison.

**Here are some good links on iron:**

https://nutritionfacts.org/topics/iron/
https://nutritionfacts.org/topics/anemia/

## Is it possible to do RT4 with diabetes?

Absolutely. Not only is it possible, a low-fat high-carb plant-based diet is proven to reverse type-2 diabetes! I've also seen many girls with type-1 diabetes who are able to greatly improve their health on this lifestyle and greatly diminish their symptoms. You'll find several members of the RT4 group who have reversed their type-2 diabetes or are easily managing their type-1.

In some cases (if you're experiencing drastic blood-sugar fluctuations, for instance) it may be important to transition into the RT4 lifestyle more slowly, rather than jumping in all at once. It is likely better for many diabetics to have several small meals throughout the day, balanced with some greens, as opposed to large fruit meals right from the start (you can work your way up to that in time). Have a salad and some steamed veggies with your dinner meal. Make sure to keep your fat intake as low as possible, ideally around 5% of total calories (this is very important). There will be some trial and error involved in determining which fruits work best for you, and for some it may be good to focus more on starches than fruit in the beginning, as the starches may be easier on blood-sugar levels while your body is still cleaning out the fat from your bloodstream. If you are currently on insulin medication, do not discontinue without informing your doctor. You will very likely need to ween yourself gradually off of your insulin, as your body begins to process sugar more efficiently.

So, if you have diabetes, before you jump straight into the lifestyle with both feet, be sure to do two things: 1. read Dr. Neal Barnard's Program for Reversing Diabetes (if you're diabetic, this is the most important book you could possibly read!) and 2. consult a health-care professional who is familiar with Dr. Barnard's work and the dietary approach to reversing diabetes, and work with them closely during your transition to a plant-based lifestyle. I'm convinced, from observing many girls, that RT4 works wonders for those with diabetes, but I also want you to be careful with serious conditions like these. Educate yourself, take your time to be sure about the steps you need to take, and be smart and careful when you do take them. But rest assured: a high carb, low fat plant based life-style is the best way to reverse type-2 diabetes.

**Links:**

https://www.pcrm.org/health/diabetes-resources/

**Samuel Barge**  3 weeks ago
Over a two year period I've gone from 318 lbs to 200 lbs on raw till 4....... Leaving alone meat and dairy was a quantum leap for me.... These videos have changed my way of thinking about food

Reply · 👍 👎

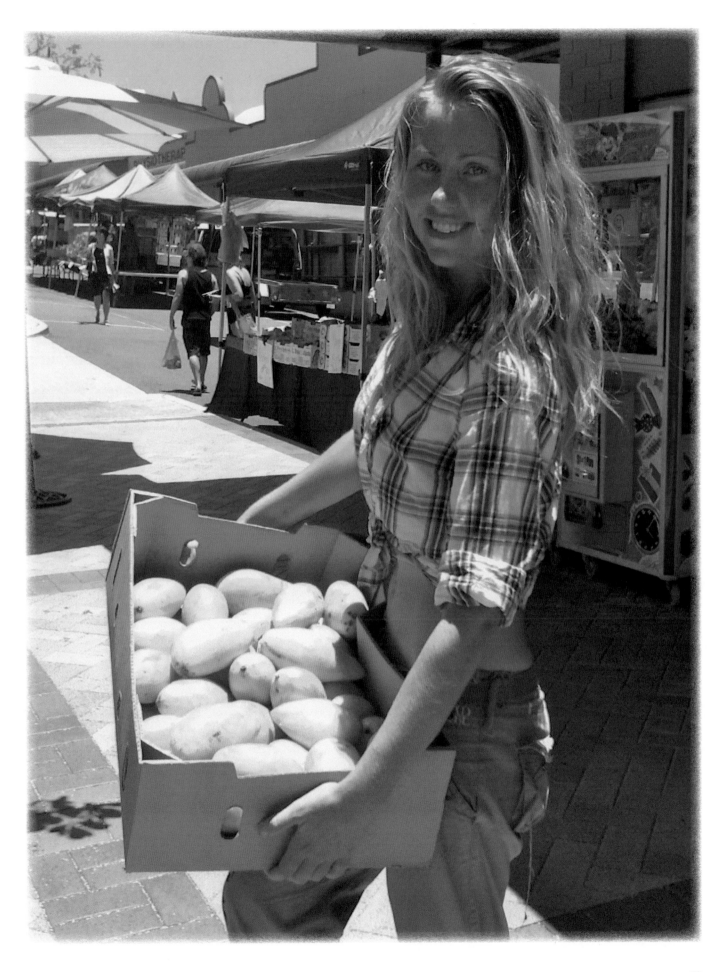

## Will this lifestyle heal my IBS, Chron's, PCOS, Hypothyroidism, etc., etc.?

Time and time again I see girls reversing these and other major health concerns on the RT4 lifestyle, so the simple answer is: yes, if you can do the lifestyle following the RT4 principles as closely as possible, and be consistent long term, there's a very good chance these and many other issues will either heal completely or diminish significantly. I for one personally healed low thyroid function (after previously being on medication).

# IBS, COLITIS & CHRON'S DISEASE

IBS and other chronic digestive issues can absolutely be cured on the RT4 lifestyle. I should know, I've done it myself! The common triggers for girls suffering with IBS are eliminated on RT4, and simply following the RT4 Principles will often bring considerable relief almost right away. The most important factors will be: keeping your fat intake low, sticking strictly to the rules of proper food combining, drinking plenty of water, getting regular exercise, adequate sleep and learning to manage stress. Though it is often claimed that fruit worsens IBS symptoms, this is only of particular concern for those following high fat diets, diets including animal products and/or combining foods incorrectly. There are certain foods to avoid, and certain rules that are important to follow while healing from IBS.

First, ripe and spotty banana smoothies are your best friend, along with soaked dates. You may enjoy adding green juices to your daily routine (not as a meal replacement though). Try celery, cucumber, spinach, and apple, add a little water and sip a cup of this daily on an empty stomach. Increase water intake between meals. Steamed veggies at night and baked sweet potato with soft tender lettuce leaves is ideal. Be sure to peel anything with a skin, like apples, potatoes, carrots, cucumbers (you can leave peels on for making the juice). Avoid any citrus, chili, onions, garlic, pepper, broccoli, cabbage, cauliflower, brussel sprouts, cruciferous greens like kale, nuts and seeds. Also be sure to eliminate spices as much as possible. It's very important to be strict on these things during the healing phase, then you can slowly reintroduce the ones you like once your digestive system is fully healed.

For those with full Chron's, it's highly recommended to focus on the simplest diet, with lots of monomeals (meal of one kind of fruit) for the first few weeks or months. You want to go as easy on your digestive system as possible. Monomeals of ripe bananas are ideal. Simple dinners of, say, sweet potato with steamed veggies, are a good option. The main idea is to give your body time to heal by focusing on the healthiest source of calories, the most easily digestible options, while minimizing or eliminating any problem foods, and being consistent. Consistency is key!

# PCOS

The first thing to know about PCOS is the difference between polycystic ovaries (where a female's ovaries contain cysts) & polycystic ovarian syndrome. For one diagnosed with PCOS, the main symptom is an irregular menstrual cycle, which is commonly accompanied by other symptoms, including acne, high or low BMI (either end of the spectrum) and abnormal hairiness. Many girls think they have PCOS when in actual fact they have polycystic ovaries but lack the other symptoms that would qualify as the full syndrome.

PCOS and polycystic ovaries are associated with hormonal imbalances, including too much of the male hormone androgen. This causes cysts to form in the ovaries, preventing them from maturing an egg and ovulating. A female with cystic ovaries can go months or years with no period or ovulation or sometimes even have 2 periods in 1 month, or extremely painful periods to the point of fainting. There are two main dangers related to this condition.

1.  When there's no menstruation, the uterus is constantly in a pre-period state (waiting to shed the blood which isn't being shed), which can lead to chronic exposure to the female hormone estrogen, along with a lack of progesterone; over the long term this imbalance increases the risk for uterine cancer (endometrial hyperplasia and carcinoma). The common gynecologist's solution is either to take the contraceptive pill or a pill called Duphaston (dydrogesterone) which you take for a period of a week to 10 days to induce bleeding (it is NOT a contraceptive).
2.  Specifically if you have the high BMI factor in combination with the other symptoms, there is a tendency to develop type-2 diabetes.

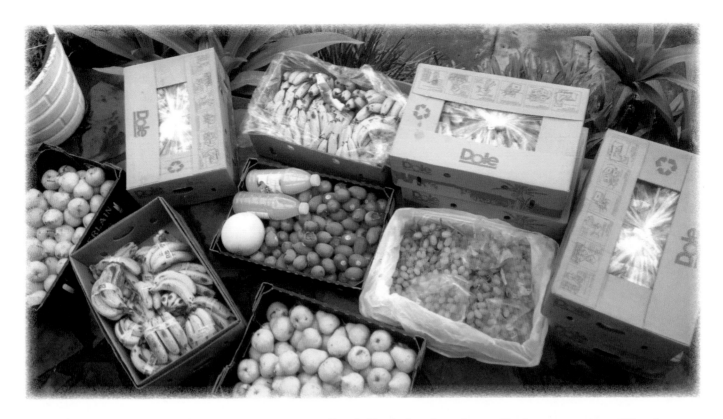

Most girls who come to RT4 with cystic ovaries or PCOS will probably also have been damaged by the contraceptive pill for a few years. Most often it's the Diane-35 pill or "Yasmin." It takes at least a year if not 2 or 3 for the body to heal itself fully from the effects of the pill, so it is important for you girls to understand that and be ready for it—it is a healing process that goes beyond the change in diet. When beginning RT4, this hormonal healing process may be accelerated, because the body is also getting all the nutrition it needs to aid/boost the process. During this time, you may expect a couple of common side effects. First, acne breakouts (these can be quite severe for some), not just on the face but also on the back, shoulders, arms, chest, neck - which I had. Second, weight gain (for girls coming from calorie restriction) or weight loss (for the obese), which will help enable regular menstruation. Initial weight fluctuation of one kind of another is to be expected, related not just to healing of your metabolism (due to adopting a healthy diet), but to healing of your hormonal system as well (due to recovering from the pill and overall rebalancing of hormone levels). It's often that the body will prioritize healing the hormonal system, particularly if it has been extremely harmed, and it can take many months, even a couple of years for it to fully rebalance. The effects from this process, including the weight fluctuation, may be added to the effects of healing that the change of diet alone may have, so girls with PCOS, and even girls who express only one or two of the symptoms commonly go through a few months of fairly strong healing processes initially. In terms of timing: some girls find that they begin to have regular menstrual cycles after only a couple of months; others within the first year of the lifestyle. Most will see significant improvements within a year. The full healing of PCOS may take longer for some.

**Key factors for healing your hormonal system are:**
1. Rest and reduced stress. Stress is a major factor, as the female menstrual cycle is VERY easily affected by stress. Don't we know it girls?
2. Cardio exercise that gets the lymphatic system moving and builds up a good sweat (recommended once per day, with a couple of rest or lower-intensity days each week).
3. Good hydration (aim to pee 8-12 times a day, clear urine)
4. Avoid all overt fats during the initial healing stage.
5. Really go for the leafy greens during the healing period; nice, big salads along with your high carb dinner is perfect.

If you give it time, stick to the RT4 lifestyle as closely as possible, PCOS can absolutely be healed/reversed on this lifestyle (the cysts can even disappear/dissolve away). I know dozens of cases of girls who have healed their PCOS, returned to a regular menstrual cycle, become fertile again, and have rebalanced their body's hormonal system fully. To put it simply: *"A plant-based diet is the best option for girls with PCOS."*—Dr. Neil Barnard

# HYPOTHYROIDISM

Most thyroid issues are significantly reduced and even removed altogether by switching to a high carb, low fat plant-based diet/lifestyle, like RT4. It has been demonstrated that vegan diets do protect against hypothyroidism, but the question is whether or not it can be reversed. The answer seems to be: it depends. It depends on the nature of the hypothyroidism (it can be caused by iodine deficiency, medications, surgery, radiation, or by "autoimmune thyroiditis" (aka Hashimoto's), where one's own immune system attacks the thyroid gland). It depends on the severity of the condition. It depends on dozens of other health questions unique to each person. So yeh, it's definitely a complex issue, overall.

What I have seen are hundreds of cases of clinically low thyroid function returning to normal levels on a high carb vegan lifestyle, both all-raw and Raw Till 4, including my own. Before this lifestyle I suffered from low thyroid function verified by a blood test and now it is perfectly balanced (also verified by a blood test). If the issue is due to low iodine especially, it should be able to be reversed with this lifestyle in no time. The other causes, and the more severe cases may not be so clear-cut. I have seen testimonials of girls who have been on medication for years (even decades!) for hypothyroidism, who feel amazing on this lifestyle and some have been able to go off their medication without symptoms returning. I have even seen a few testimonials of diagnosed autoimmune thyroiditis (Hashimoto's) being reversed on the lifestyle. For now, we can say that this lifestyle definitely improves thyroid function, and will reverse many thyroid issues. In serious cases of hypothyroidism it is still advisable to work closely with a doctor (preferably a vegan-friendly doctor) to track how the lifestyle may be improving the issue, and determine together if medication is still required.

## Will this lifestyle help me get my period back?

Firstly, it's important to understand that Raw Till 4 is a healing lifestyle and everyone will go through a period (no pun intended) of healing and detox. Starting a healthy, high carb vegan lifestyle will, for most of us, begin a hormonal healing process. I know it did for me. It's difficult to anticipate exactly how the process will go for each individual, because each is coming from a unique health background. But there are two common scenarios that we can touch on here.

1. Coming to the lifestyle with no period and getting it back.
2. Coming to the lifestyle with a period, losing it at the beginning of the lifestyle, and then gaining it back after your body has healed.

### For the first scenario:

Coming to this lifestyle with no period can be a result of a few things: 1. a background of calorie restriction and low BMI, which can disrupt or eliminate one's menstruation, 2. PCOS (see response on PCOS), and several other reasons, which may be unknown/undiagnosed, one example being the consumption of animal products, which can aggravate P.M.S. and cause irregularity in one's cycle.

If you have issues during menstruation, or no menstruation at all, adopting a high carb, low fat, vegan lifestyle will most definitely help you. If you make sure you eat enough! This lifestyle has been demonstrated to be ideal for regulation of our body's hormonal systems, and I've seen many girls who have been able to restore a balanced, healthy reproductive system, without the aid of any kind of medication.

If you were calorie restricting, and are now following the RT4 Principles, your body may gain some short-term weight—one thing this allows is the ability to rebalance your hormone system and allow regular menstruation to occur again. In these situations it may be that the hormonal healing will be prioritized, so that your body may not begin to fully normalize its BMI until the hormonal healing has had a chance to reach a certain point of progress. This is entirely natural. Another common symptom that can arise during the healing process is acne. Some will experience acne breakouts, usually on their face, shoulders, back or arms. I also experienced this although I was coming from a past of acne as well. These are both part of the balancing process and will clear up in time. It can be difficult to deal with acne breakouts and weight gain, so definitely reach out to those who have gone through it for support and encouragement. If you're experiencing this scenario, try to just stick to the RT4 Principles as closely as you can, be patient, trust in your body, and allow it to rebalance your hormonal system. Then you can celebrate the return of your body to its full glory!

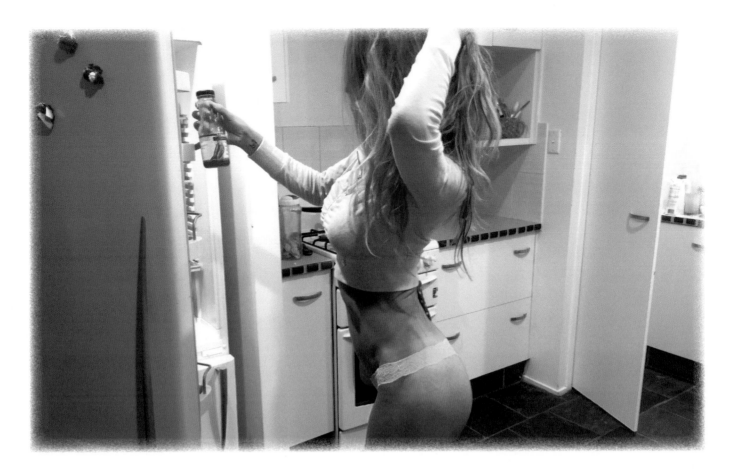

## For the second scenario:

Girls' who come to this lifestyle will be healing anything from diabetes to digestive illnesses to PCOS, or even cancer or overcoming damage
from the contraceptive pill. The most common issues to heal among females are the results of eating disorders, calorie restriction and yo-yo dieting. So with all this healing going on, it's no wonder some girls's bodies may suspend the full effects of menstruation for a while. There are priorities in our bodily mechanisms, and a full and healthy menstrual cycle can be a lower priority than some other internal healing if that healing is vitally important. Think about it this way, your body is going to put your reproductive cycle on the back-burner until it's got the rest of you sorted out, because reproducing is the last thing on the to-do-list when a lot of healing is taking place. This suspension can last from a couple of months to more than a year, depending on many factors (each person's journey will be totally unique in this regard).

It can really stress us if we lose our period, and it's not uncommon to freak out a little when that happens! But we must remember the human body's amazing ability to heal itself, and educate ourselves on what missing our period can mean. In the end, the best thing is to relax, enjoy the holiday, and allow your body to heal at its own pace. There is a chance, of course, that you're pregnant, so it's always a good idea to check that first. When I came to the raw vegan lifestyle back in 2007 I lost my period for 9 months, it felt right at the time. I was healing from over 7 years of taking the contraceptive pill. Today my period is light and mostly painless, certainly nothing like it used to be!

Losing your period (amenorrhea), can also occur when weight and/or body fat % is dramatically low. If this may be your case, it's important to address it as soon as possible. Just focus on the RT4 Principles, especially on getting in enough carbohydrate calories. PLEASE DON'T STARVE YOURSELF. This is a lifestyle of abundance and your body will thank you long term.

Even though you have lost your period you may still experience some of the common symptoms like cramps, mood swings, cravings; this is a sign that you are still ovulating and menstruating. Irregular, really long periods, or losing it entirely are most often signs of hormonal imbalances which will balance out on this lifestyle in time if you can follow the RT4 Principles closely. Most importantly keep the fat low and the carbs high!

## What to expect in terms of menstruation on the RT4 lifestyle:

As well as balancing out hormones, Raw Till 4 has many other positive benefits regarding that time of the month. Most girls who follow Raw Till 4 and other low fat, low protein, high carb lifestyles experience one or more of these benefits:

1. Less period pain/cramps or none at all
2. Lighter periods
3. Shorter periods (2-4 days)
4. More stable moods and less or no cravings.

*I experienced all 4 plus more. I used to regularly skip days off work to rock in the corner hugging my legs in pain. :(*

In general, girls on RT4 will experience periods that are shorter, less painful with lighter flow. Most girls report that they come to feel much more at ease with their cycle; it's not as strong, not as disruptive when it happens, it doesn't smack them in the face quite so hard. Some long term RT4 girls, who are physically fit and in optimal health, may experience little to no bleeding but still be ovulating. In this case, it's important to know that even if you aren't experiencing bleeding it's still possible to get pregnant. It's also possible to menstruate each month but not be actively ovulating. So it's important to understand that having or not having your period is not the same as ovulating or not ovulating. You may want to see a gynaecologist/endocrinologist to confirm which applies to you. Be aware of the natural consequences of having sex, regardless of which stage of this journey you're on. Be safe, smart and know your body. Girls, definitely encourage your partner to get a vasectomy then you can have worry-free sex. It will change both your lives for the better.

It's crucial to keep fat and protein low (below 10%, close to 5%) during your period in order to reap the best benefits when it comes to your menstrual cycle. It can also be very helpful to increase your caloric intake (even by as much as 1000 calories) as this time of the month can be taxing on energy. So don't be afraid to carb up even more than usual! Remember to eat unlimited high carb plant foods, as well as drinking 3+ litres of water to keep your blood and body strong and healthy.

## A little more on the topic:

I recommend you invest in alternatives to traditional sanitary items such as menstrual cups, ask me for recommendations. Myself and many others have found that their period pains reduce after switching to using menstrual cups. These methods are free of toxins and much friendlier on the environment. There are also reusable washable pads if you're not into menstrual cups (see my video link below for more info on menstrual cups).

The contraceptive pill interferes with the body's natural hormone regulation and rhythms and can, among other things, increase risk of blood clots. Many girls choose to stop taking the pill along their health journey. This can be a large contributing factor towards having an irregular cycle or losing it all together for a while, as it can take up to a couple of years for the body to fully rebalance after going off the pill. Another common symptom of going off the pill is weight fluctuation (either weight loss or weight gain), as weight (especially water retention, etc.) is impacted directly by hormones. Reactions like these are normal considering the body has been taking in mixtures of hormones every day for extended periods of time and is now rebalancing.

## Here is a video I made that you may find helpful:

Menstrual Cups, I Love Them, My Tips, by Freelee: http://youtu.be/NHniznqJtBE

**Tara Robinson**  1 day ago
+Katiemakesfaces I feel the same way!!!  I struggled with eating disorders too now I don't worry how many calories I eat.  As long as I got my fruit and smoothies,  I'm good! No more binges on junk food.  I'm so happy.  I've lost 13 pounds and my skin is clearing up!  I'm so happy I found freelee <3

Reply · 1 👍 👎

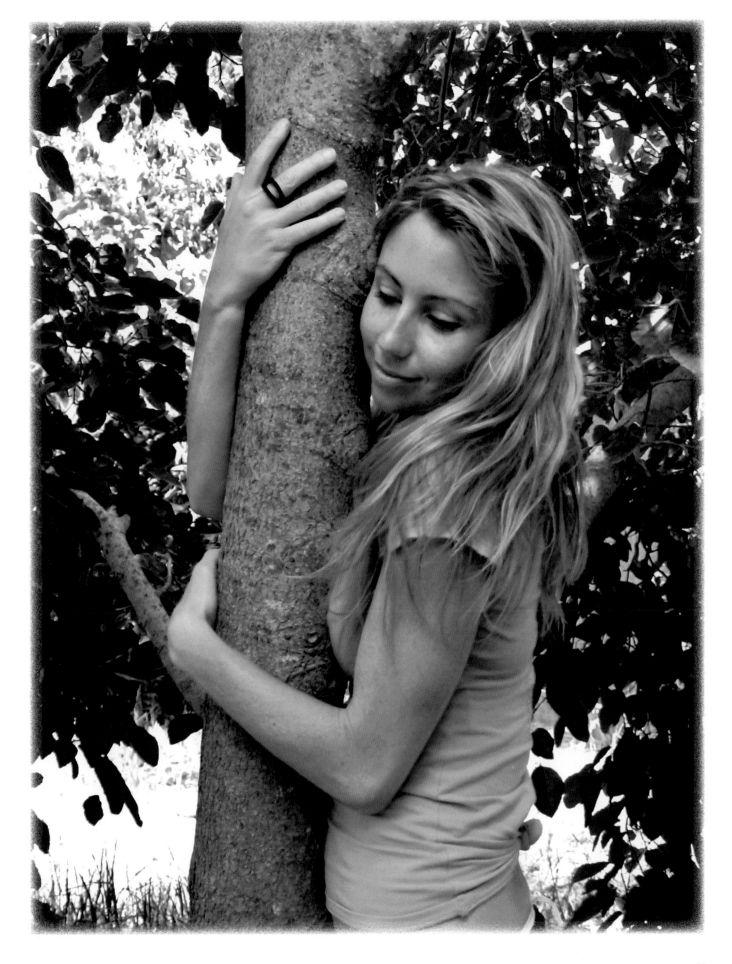

# INGREDIENTS AND FOOD COMBINING

## *What about gluten?*

It's definitely a controversial topic. Some say there is not such thing as gluten-intolerance, others suffer after consuming it. I, for one, find that I tolerate small amounts of gluten but not large amounts. So I find I do much better on a low-no gluten diet.

A little less than 1% of the population have celiac disease, a full intolerance (inability to digest) gluten. For these girls, gluten must be completely avoided. For all others, there may be no need to completely eliminate gluten, but there may be reasons to minimize the amount of gluten one includes in their diet. It may also be important for girls who are healing from digestive issues to avoid gluten entirely until they've healed themselves of those issues. It's also important to keep in mind that girls rarely eat gluten-containing foods clean: they're usually also loaded with fat, covered in dairy, and other junk. Thus, many of the health issues commonly associated with gluten are likely actually caused by animal products and oils. This is super important to keep in mind. Doctors like Dr. McDougall and Dr. Greger, and plant-based nutritionists like Suzan Levin, stand by the position that for anyone who is non-celiac, gluten is actually ok for you, and is fine to play a role in your high carb vegan diet.

### Links: (type into your browser)
https://www.drmcdougall.com/misc/2013nl/mar/gluten.htm
http://nutritionfacts.org/video/is-gluten-bad-for-you/
http://nutritionfacts.org/video/update-on-gluten/

It seems, however, that gluten may help cause and exasperate certain digestive illnesses and an array of autoimmune diseases that essentially begin in the gut. The key issue seems to be gluten's role in triggering the protein zonulin, which is the "doorway" to Leaky Gut Syndrome (see the research done by Dr. Fasano). Leaky Gut means that the intestinal wall has become more porous, allowing molecules into the bloodstream that wouldn't normally make their way in so easily. Once in the bloodstream, these can cause all kinds of autoimmune issues as the body tries to fight off these intruders. In order to heal, one needs to remove the foods that were causing the issue, which will mean removing all animal products, oils, and apparently gluten as well, while focusing on as clean a diet as possible. Once one's digestive system has healed one may be able to include small amounts of gluten in one's diet without suffering negative effects, but that will be for each to determine for themselves. Gluten may also play a role as a neurotoxin that can cause damage to nerve tissue—many girls with neurological diseases (autism, migraine headaches, ADD, bipolar, schizophrenia, neuropathy, epilepsy, etc.) have been shown to do well on a gluten free diet.

On the RT4 lifestyle, gluten need not play a primary role anyway; it's naturally a fairly gluten-free lifestyle. If you focus on our recommended starch staples (rice, potatoes, corn, etc.) then you'll be more-or-less gluten free anyway. Gluten will come into play for things like wraps or perhaps the occasional vegan pizza or small amounts of mock-meats on very rare occasions. Gluten is in some pre-made sauces, gravies, etc., as well, but those are also only occasional foods on this lifestyle. Most long term RT4ers tend not to consume much gluten even without making a strict effort to avoid it. So RT4 makes no strict rule against gluten, but does recommend not to make gluten-containing foods part of your main staples: minimize gluten when you can for the most optimal results.

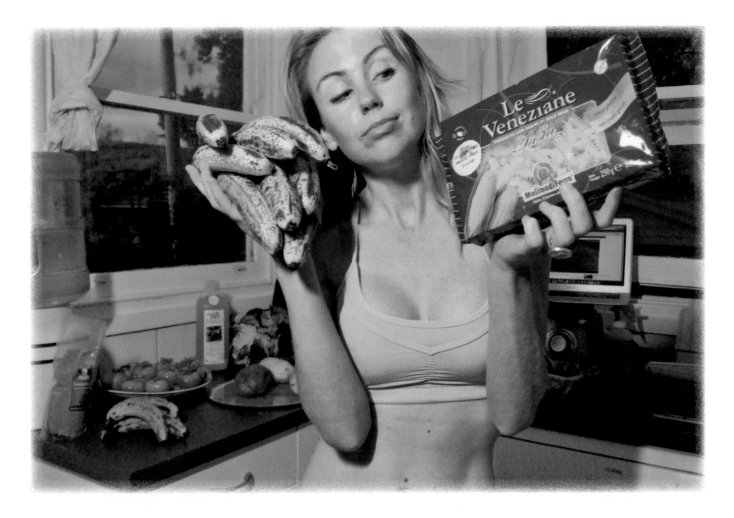

## What about almond milk, chia seeds, flax, popcorn, soy, etc...?

The Raw Till 4 lifestyle is intended to be one of abundance, and particularly one of an abundance of clean, healthy, high energy carb-loaded foods. The primary focus should always be on consuming adequate amounts of healthy carbohydrates at each and every meal. Simply put, you always want to be carbed-up! Though popcorn, and other low-calorie dry foods like popped lotus seeds and rice crackers, are fine, they're actually pretty empty foods. They offer little in the way of carbohydrates and calories, they are often dehydrating and sometimes even difficult to digest. Many girls tend to feel the need to "dress" these foods in any number of toppings that often include high-fat and high-sodium contents, which will only hamper your results on this lifestyle. These foods provide minimal nutrition or energy and yet they can easily fill your tummy. This can then take the place of healthy, nutrient-dense and energizing plant foods that could and should be eaten instead. Essentially, low-carb foods and low-cal foods like popcorn offer very little payoff for the body. They're ok as snacks, but always make sure they're not interfering with your ability to eat enough of the RT4 staple foods. Foods like almond milk fall into the same category as other high-fat vegan foods: they're ok here and there for sure, but are best avoided as staples.

Many modern nutritionists and doctors (like Dr. Greger, for instance) recommend chia seeds, flax seeds, nuts and other seeds in order to help meet our daily needs of omega-3, because the science does show these foods to have some beneficial and disease fighting properties. However, on the RT4 lifestyle, when one is not consuming health-damaging foods like meat and dairy or lots of oils, the same beneficial properties are obtained simply from an abundance of high carbohydrate fruits and starches. On RT4, I recommend to limit these foods in the same way I recommend to limit other higher fat foods. They're ok once and a while, but not necessary for overall health on this lifestyle. Eat them if you wish, but try to keep your daily fat intake low. Definitely no need to make these foods regular staples. Low fat (under 10% of total calories) is the idea for optimal long term health as a high carb vegan.

# EXERCISE

Being fit is really important to our quality of life. If we desire all round health, then we must move our butts regularly! The animal in nature that doesn't move daily, doesn't eat, and eventually dies. We are designed to move and play. Our lymphatic system needs to be pumped often to eliminate waste, and our cells require large quantities of fresh ozygen daily. Physical activity stimulates energy consumption and the secretion of important feel good hormones that mobilise fat deposits for elimiation. Exercise regulates blood sugar levels so we feel balanced. It optimises nutrient absorption and assimilation. Personally, running and cycling are my favourite forms of play. I recommend you grab a Garmin watch to time and pace yourself. How much intensity for running? It depends on what you are trying to achieve and what your current fitness level is. Every workout should start with a thorough warm up.

Walk briskly for 5-10 minutes before jogging. If you find your basic running routine I have included too easy then please take out the rest periods, or step it up to the intermediate program. Please be conservative with your running training. It is EASY to become injured if you area newbie to running. I've included the following beginner fitness program with is BASIC and repetitive for a reason, your tendons, ligaments, joints, bones, and muscles need time to adapt to the increased impact. If you feel any joint pain then please power walk instead.

Go in as many running races as you can, even if you just walk it! I know the sound of a running race may be daunting, but it is worth it trust me. Running races have improved my self-esteem and body dramatically over the years. Join up to your local park run, they are free, you can google more details. Over the next 30 days I challenge you to find a running race you can sign up for. My mum is over 60 and she goes in them and jog/walks. No excuses! Find one in your local area and get it girls! First up though, lets talk about my current love - cycling!

## HOW I BECAME A BANANAGIRLBIKER

I first go into cycling in 2008. I ended up selling my car, bought a bicycle and rode solo across Australia over 3000kms! I wanted to challenge myself both physically and mentally and I certainly did that. This made me realise just how cool cycling actually was! Over the years I gradually got fitter, lost weight and became a much happier person largely from the inclusion of regular cycling and jogging. Now it's time for me to share all my cycling motivation and tips with you Banana Girls. You may be like 'ugh do I HAVE to get a bike?' Well yes, if you want to get the fastest results then cycling enables you to transform your metabolism into a serious fat-burner. Invest short term and receive the long term gains. Get a bike between your legs girl!

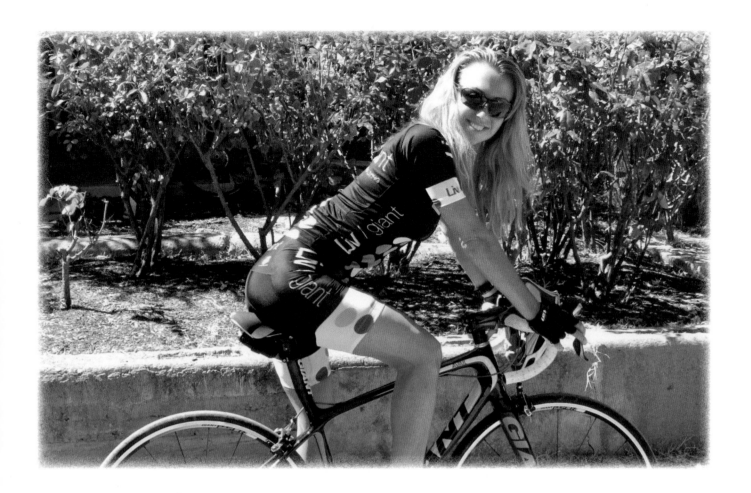

# BIKE RECOMMENDATIONS AND FITTING

Giant brand bikes are my bike of choice. Specifically Giant Avail Series, which one exactly depends on your budget. I have tried just about every other brand and find they do not measure up to a Giant. It's important to get your bike fitted up to you. A good bike fit is really important for comfort and performance. Make sure you get the shop to give you a bike fit before you leave the store. Mark all your measurements with a white out pen - seat height, saddle angle/fore/aft, cleat position, handlebar angle etc.

**Banana Girl Biker Accessories:**
- Invest in a Garmin to track your km's and effort. Which one depends on your budget. I use the Garmin 1000 because it has maps.
- Sign up to **www.strava.com** and log your rides. It's a free fitness tracking app and you may just meet a fit vegan guy on there.

**Banana Girl Bike Safety:**
- When overtaking a parked car always leave enough room for the driver to swing their door out. It's a good idea to signal slightly with your hand to the car behind that you are coming out.
- Ride at least a metre away from the edge of the road where it drops away to gravel even if you feel like you are in the way of the traffic. If you don't do this cars will try to push along side you and possibly cause you to go into the gravel and lose your balance.
- Always wear cycling gloves to protect your hands from gravel rash incase you fall off.
- Of course ALWAYS wear a helmet, it may just save your life one day.
- Even though it is the law in many countries, as a baby Banana Girl I recommend you avoid riding two abreast and stick to single file.
- As a newbie, avoid riding in groups or ride at the back of groups.
- Be confident in the traffic as this will help the driver have confidence in your movements. Unpredictable riders are a danger on the road.

# BANANA GIRL BIKING

Not only will you be overhauling how you eat, but also how you move. I wouldn't be as fit, lean and healthy as I am without a consistent bike routine. The 7 day example below is designed to be very easy to follow and implement. The more complicated an exercise routine the less likely you are to stick to it in the long term. Below is just a 7 day example:

**DAY 1:** Ride at a comfortable talking pace on the flat for 20 mins
**DAY 2:** Ride at a comfortable talking pace on the flat for 20 mins
**DAY 3:** Find a slight incline/hill and ride up it a few times or until you reach 10 mins
**DAY 4:** REST
**DAY 5:** Ride at a comfortable talking pace on the flat for 20 mins
**DAY 6:** Find a slight incline/hill and ride up it a few times or until you reach 10 mins
**DAY 7:** REST

It really is THAT simple, increase the time, distance, intensity as you go and have fun!

# JOGGING FOR FITNESS

Something I don't do as much now that I have a bike is jogging. However, I still recommend it as a great form of exercise for those who already have a good fitness base. Please remember that jogging can be particularly hard on your joints so you need to be conservative in your approach. If you have a significant amount of excess weight to release then I recommend you bike ride instead of jog. Below are some of my best tips and on the following page is a beginner and intermediate jogging routine to get you started!

**Jogging tips:**
- Invest in some quality running shoes that provide support. Barefoot running would be ideal but with hard surfaces commonplace, I don't recommend it.
- Make sure you are hydrated with plenty of clean water before you jog, and get plenty afterwards. Aim to be peeing clear at least 8-10 times per day.
- Warm up and cool down with at least 5 mins of walking.
- Imagine you are holding butterflies/ripe figs in your palms as you run, this helps discourage clenching your fists too tightly. Keep nipples facing forward, hands low, arms held at right angles swinging by your sides and not across your body. Avoid swinging your whole upper boy, as this movement travels down to your lower body subsequently affecting your foot strike, which can lead to injury.
- Do yoga (salutes to the sun) stretching after your jog, or some other dynamic stretching routine.

*On the following pages you will find a basic and intermediate running program. Please listen to your body and don't overdo it!*

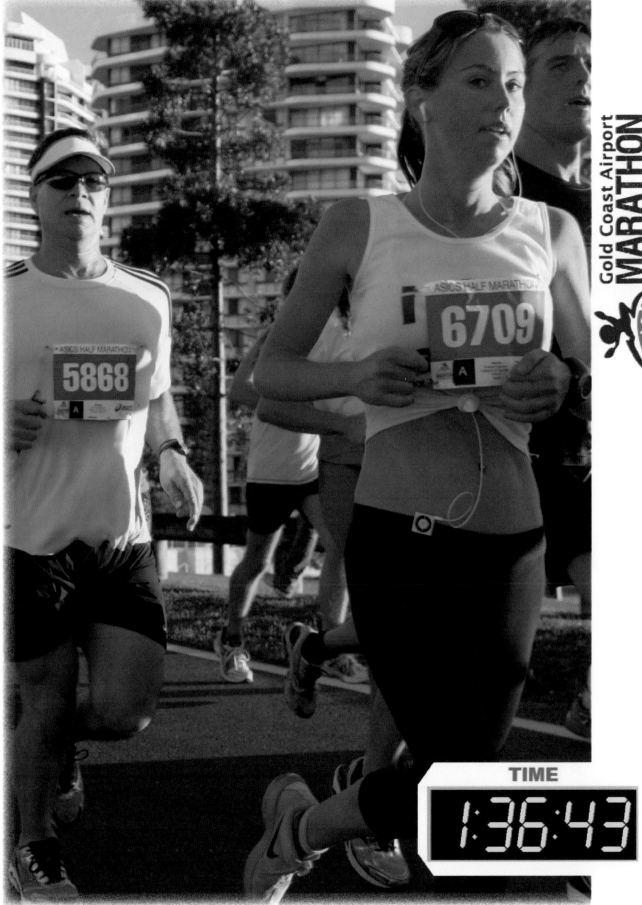

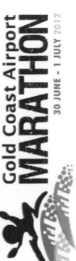

Gold Coast Airport
MARATHON
30 JUNE – 1 JULY 2012

ASICS HALF MARATHON
5868
A

ASICS HALF MARATHON
6709
A

TIME
1:36:43

# 30 DAYS OF PLAY (BEGINNER)

" If you find this routine too easy then take out the rest periods. Please be conservative with your running training. It is EASY to become injured if you are a newbie. This program is BASIC and repetitive for a reason. Your tendons, ligaments, joints, bones, and muscles need time to adapt to the increased impact. If you feel any joint pain then please power walk instead. Most of all have fun and enjoy the runners high! Please warm up for 5-10 mins before and after this routine. "

|  | WEEK 1 | WEEK 2 | WEEK 3 | WEEK 4 |
|---|---|---|---|---|
| **DAY 1** | jog at easy pace for 2 mins then walk for 80 secs **REPEAT PROCESS FOR TOTAL 15 MINS** | jog at easy pace for 2.30 mins then walk for 80 secs **REPEAT PROCESS FOR TOTAL 20 MINS** | jog at easy pace for 3 mins then walk for 80 secs. Jog for 4 mins then walk for 80 secs **REPEAT** | jog at easy pace for 5 mins then walk for 80 secs **REPEAT PROCESS 3-4 TIMES** |
| **DAY 2** | jog at easy pace for 2 mins then walk for 80 secs **REPEAT PROCESS FOR TOTAL 15 MINS** | jog at easy pace for 2.30 mins then walk for 80 secs **REPEAT PROCESS FOR TOTAL 20 MINS** | jog at easy pace for 3 mins then walk for 80 secs. Jog for 4 mins then walk for 80 secs **REPEAT** | jog at easy pace for 5 mins then walk for 80 secs **REPEAT PROCESS 3-4 TIMES** |
| **DAY 3** | jog at easy pace for 2 mins then walk for 80 secs **REPEAT PROCESS FOR TOTAL 15 MINS** | jog at easy pace for 2.30 mins then walk for 80 secs **REPEAT PROCESS FOR TOTAL 20 MINS** | jog at easy pace for 3 mins then walk for 80 secs. Jog for 4 mins then walk for 80 secs **REPEAT** | jog at easy pace for 5 mins then walk for 80 secs **REPEAT PROCESS 3-4 TIMES** |
| **DAY 4** | Cross-train! preferably jump on your bike and ride **FOR AT LEAST 30 MINS** | Cross-train! preferably jump on your bike and ride **FOR AT LEAST 30 MINS** | Cross-train! preferably jump on your bike and ride **FOR AT LEAST 30 MINS** | Cross-train! preferably jump on your bike and ride **FOR AT LEAST 30 MINS** |

- On the days that aren't included, please rest or walk
- Easy pace means you should be able to maintain a conversation

# 30 DAYS OF PLAY (ADVANCED)

" This is an intermediate to advanced running routine. I don't recommend you do this routine if you are new to running. Several months of adaption must take place before you commence this routine. Please warm up sufficiently by joging easy for 5-10 mins first. You will really benefit from having a Garmin watch to track your pace. Listen to your body for injuries and most importantly enjoy! "

|  | WEEK 1 | WEEK 2 | WEEK 3 | WEEK 4 |
|---|---|---|---|---|
| **DAY 1** | Hill repeats. Run at 80% of your max effort up a med size hill for 30 secs walk/jog down. **REPEAT x10** | **CROSSTRAIN** or Rest | Hill repeats. Run at 80% of your max effort up a med size hill for 30 secs walk/jog down. **REPEAT x12** | Intervals: After warm up run 500 mtrs at your race pace or faster, 1 min recovery. **REPEAT x5** |
| **DAY 2** | Moderate pace jog for **45 MINS** | **LSD - LONG SLOW DISTANCE** 1 hr 20 mins. Run at conversational pace, good for building endurance | Moderate pace jog for **45 MINS** | **CROSSTRAIN** or Rest |
| **DAY 3** | Cross-train! preferably jump on your bike and ride **FOR AT LEAST 30 MINS** | Moderate pace jog for **45 MINS** | Intervals: After warm up run 500 mtrs at your race pace or faster, 1 min recovery. **REPEAT x5** | Hill repeats. Run at 80% of your max effort up a med size hill for 30 secs walk/jog down. **REPEAT x12** |
| **DAY 5** | **LSD - LONG SLOW DISTANCE** 1 hr 20 mins. Run at conversational pace, good for building endurance | Hill repeats. Run at 80% of your max effort up a med size hill for 30 secs walk/jog down. **REPEAT x10** | Rest or crosstrain! Preferably jump on your bike and ride for at least **30 MINS** | Moderate pace jog for **45 MINS** |
| **DAY 6** | Intervals: After warm up run 500 mtrs at your race pace or faster, 1 min recovery. **REPEAT x5** | Rest or crosstrain! Preferably jump on your bike and ride for at least **30 MINS** | **LSD - LONG SLOW DISTANCE** 1 hr 20 mins. Run at conversational pace, good for building endurance | Rest or crosstrain! Preferably jump on your bike and ride for at least **30 MINS** |

- Moderate pace means maintaining a conversation is difficult
- During short hill bursts and intervals you should not be physically able to talk

# MISCELLANEOUS

## What if I want to be fully raw?

After many years being 100% raw, I've moved away from recommending a fully raw lifestyle simply because for the majority of girls it proves to be unsustainable. If, however, you're in a life-situation where abundant ripe fruit is available year round, and you have the time, money and passion to stick to it, a fully raw lifestyle can be very healthy. However, over time our experience is that the results on RT4 are largely the same, if not a little better, than on a fully raw vegan lifestyle, so I don't want anyone to feel pressure that they need to be all-raw. Some fully raw proponents will have you believe it's easy peasy but it really isn't. Sure if you have a personal chef, a huge budget and endless high quality fruit on tap!

The first thing to do if you want to aim to be raw vegan is to get my first ebook "**Go Fruit Yourself**". It chronicles the beginning of my high carb raw vegan lifestyle, demonstrating all the common mistakes and helping you to see the critical points of how to make the lifestyle healthy and sustainable. The number one point is to get enough calories daily! The number one reason girls fail at a fully raw lifestyle long term, is failing to eat enough.

## SUPERFOODS, TONICS AND EXTRACTS

"Superfood" is one of the biggest buzzwords in the health-industry. It's also one of the biggest scams. Diet isn't a chemistry experiment, and your body doesn't need to be a lab. People who sell you superfoods want you to think that you need some specific extract or tonic because it has some specific vitamin or mineral (or woo-woo magic) in it, but whole fresh fruits have all the vitamins and minerals we need from dietary sources, all in one package. If we're eating the right diet and living a healthy lifestyle we don't need any extra "superfoods." Fruit is the best superfood on the planet!

Remember that the body is holistic; all we need to do is provide it with the right conditions and it'll thrive. It doesn't need us to spend thousands of dollars on strange and exotic potions in order to function properly. The RT4 lifestyle doesn't include any "superfoods," or extracts, or tonics, or pills or potions. Be free of all that. Save your money for bananas, dates, bikes, trips and for enjoying life!

## How do you afford the RT4 lifestyle?

It's quite easy, actually. The key is to focus on the cheapest, most abundantly available fruits and starches as your main staples. Bananas are the staple fruit for most RT4ers, and they're typically cheap and available just about anywhere. Rice, potatoes and corn are among the cheapest foods on the planet and can form your main dinner staples. Use these as your staples and it'll be easily affordable. Then, feast on seasonal fruits and veggies to add variety, and play around with as many dinner recipes as you can to find the ones you love.

Another helpful key to making this lifestyle affordable, especially for couples or families, is to learn to buy certain foods in bulk. Rice, pastas, etc., especially. Also bananas, dates, mangos, etc. See if you can find these in bulk at discounts. Talk to your local produce managers to build up relationships, seek out farmer's markets. Become a smart and conscientious grocery shopper, and that part of this lifestyle quickly becomes easy and enjoyable.

# But you're not a Doctor Freelee!

In an age when the whole of human knowledge is at our fingertips, the most important thing for everyone who is trying to be healthier is to do your own research. That's what I've done, and that's what I want you to do. I don't want anyone to just blindly take my word for it. However, I do want to help you avoid the years of trial-and-error that many of us went through in our health journeys, by presenting you with as much good information as I can. I want you to verify for yourselves not only that a high carb plant-based diet works, but why it works.

Although I do have advanced certification in nutrition, the information I acquired is outdated and just plain inaccurate. Years of experience coaching thousands of girls is a FAR more important credential than a piece of paper you can pay for. That said, you will still find plenty of professionals recommending the same fundamental principles of health as I do: high carb, low fat, low protein, vegan, with exercise, plenty of water, regular sleep cycles, low stress, and a focus on whole fresh foods like fruit, starches and veggies. There's no secret there, really. All I've done is take those principles, apply them to my life and experimented until I've come to what I believe to be the most optimal lifestyle principles.

## To begin your research, try starting here:

https://www.pcrm.org/
https://nutritionfacts.org/
https://www.drmcdougall.com/
https://nutritionstudies.org/
https://www.thechinastudy.com/
https://www.nealbarnard.org/
https://www.forksoverknives.com/

One other note on the subject of credentials: it's important to understand that conventional doctors are NOT taught any more than the most basic nutrition; most are absolutely unqualified to give nutritional advice. In addition to this, as far as medical or nutritional schooling goes, it takes years for new discoveries, even when proven beyond a shadow of a doubt, to make their way into the curriculum. This means that most people with certifications have been educated based on old, and very often outdated information, and unless they take the initiative to educate themselves outside of school and their career, they are just as likely to be misinformed as any average person with access to Google.

Here's a quote from Dr. Caldwell Esselstyn on the subject. It's drawn from his response when asked the question: **"why don't Doctor's promote plant-based nutrition?"**

*"It's been estimated that it takes about 17 years for new information that has been found to get into the clinical arena. I think now though, with the internet and other things, it'll happen more rapidly. I think that as we have outcomes that are so powerful, it's going to be very very hard for clinicians not to employ this [plant-based diet as a healing modality]. But there's a problem though: clinicians like to be compensated for their time spent with patients. Right now, insurance companies are not paying the physicians for the time spent doing this [investigating/practicing dietary methods of healing], so it's much more [financially] rewarding for physicians to hand out pills, to do procedures ... so compensation is a factor. ... but you're talking now about behavioural modification and you're talking about nutrition, and most of the doctors have no knowledge in that arena. So they either have to school themselves to obtain this knowledge, or they've got to relinquish the patient, send them to somebody else, who does have the skillset to help these patients."*

Let's put this in perspective. The internet is only 25 years old. Nutritional research takes about 17 years to make it into the clinical arena. This means that the information currently being taught to clinicians all around the world dates to a time when the internet still used dial-up connections! Furthermore, it's not only a question of how long it takes for information to get into the curriculum, it's a question of bias against good science when it counters girls's deeply held beliefs and/or when it counters vested interests or threatens the mighty dollar (pharmaceuticals, surgeries, etc., along with animal agriculture, are BIG businesses; do not underestimate their ability to drive policy in the field of health and nutrition). The findings of the China Study, for instance, was compiled in the mid 1980s, published in peer reviewed journals, and stand as a monumental (and life-changing) information in the field of nutrition. It's findings, however, have yet to make it into the standard curriculum. On the other hand, the belief that humans need protein from animal products continues to form the core of most clinicians personal belief systems and personal lifestyle choices.

It's for these, and many other reasons, that I constantly repeat that if you want to find health, follow those who are getting the results you desire. Credentials mean nothing if the person who has them cannot keep themselves healthy. If a doctor is obese, why take their advice on nutrition? If a nutritionist is recommending milk or eggs or other foods overwhelmingly demonstrated to be unhealthy, why take their advice? Do your own research, become your own guide, lead yourself to health. That's the key. Look into the science, the most up-to-date science, and simultaneously look into those who are getting the results you desire—when you find the science matching the lifestyle of those people, then you'll know you've got the answer!

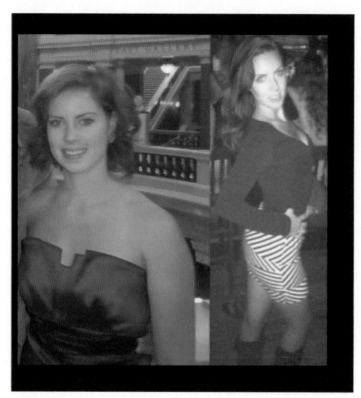

OMGEE Freelee eating Raw til 4 made me gain weight! You're such a lair 😊

Unlike · Comment

 Freelee the Banana Girl, Ken Lee, Sam Simons, Abi Evans and 29 others like this.

💬 View 1 more comment

Joanna Kingsbury Vegetarian for 8 years tried to be vegan but failed. I restricted calories, exercised like crazy and 8 years later was convinced I needed to eat meat and dairy. Eating animals and dairy was horrible - I gained weight and got crazy acne. After a year of doing that I had enough. I went 100% vegan and connected again with my old ethnics. I started to feel much better but I still ate high processed vegan food. For the last six months I have been almost processed food free and eating Raw til 4! I love it so much! And my acne has improved. I'm not perfect though and I'm always improving but this is a lifestyle you really have to stick with! I found you and Durian about a year ago and you both have helped so much through my transition. Overall since my transition I have lost 25 lbs. Its taken a long time though to not yo-yo up and down with my weight. The biggest lesson I have learned is to eat, eat eat and carb the fuck up!
August 29 at 9:14am · Unlike · 👍 12

 Ashlea Murphy I highly recommend Raw till 4, I was an 'under weight' anorexic. To the point where even now I still have to check into hospital once a week to make sure im not going backwards. It got to the point I was told I cant have children and my bones are now brittle. I turned to RT4 as my last chance of beating anorexia. Well my doctors LOVE this lifestyle, they think it is brilliant. My blood test have shown a huge improvement im now not in danger of organ failure and my hormones have shown slight improvement. Overall ive become so healthy. And yes I gained 10kg yet ive stayed slim. In the past when ive gained weight under doctors guide I put on a lot of fat and got chunky. Freelee the Banana Girl I just want you to know you are the reason im alive today.
Unlike · Reply · 👍 74 · Yesterday at 11:04am · Edited

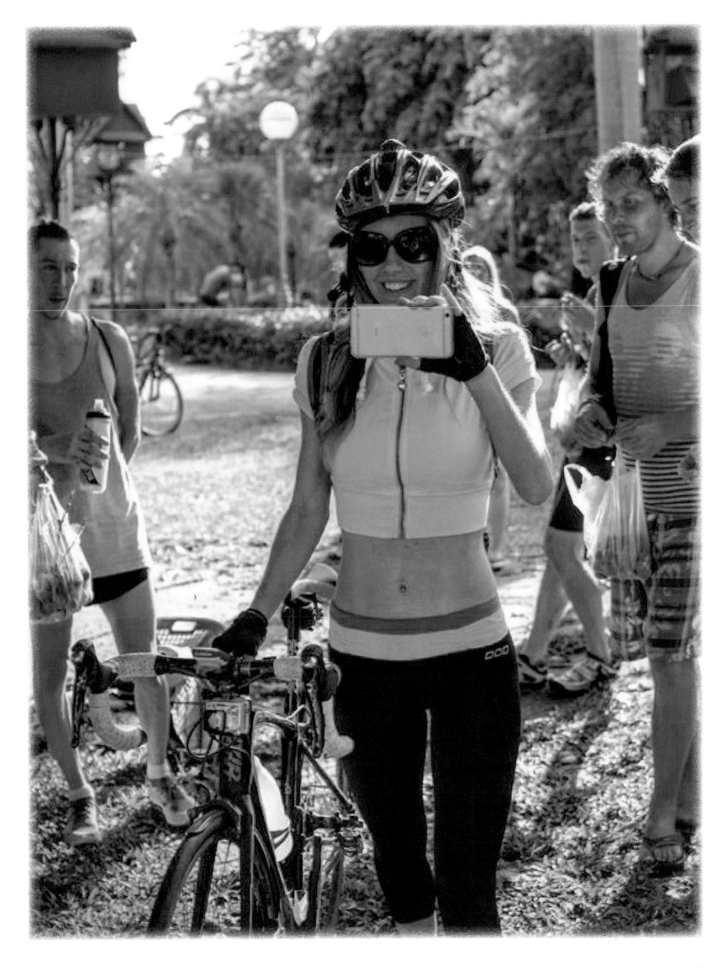

# AM I HYDRATED?

## URINE COLOR CHART

If your urine matches these 3 colors,
you are properly hydrated.
Continue to drink water to
maintain this hydration level.

If your urine colour is below the **RED LINE**
you are **DEHYDRATED**
and at risk of cramping,
slowed metabolism, and serious conditions
associated with heat illnes.

## YOU NEED TO DRINK MORE WATER!

Please aim to be drinking
enough water so you are peeing clear
8-12 times a day.

R A W T I L L 4

# RAW TILL 4 FOOD PYRAMID

**Women:** Min of 2100 calories, 2500+ to really thrive!
**Men:** Min of 2500 calories, 3000+ to really thrive!
*BUY ORGANIC WHENEVER POSSIBLE

 If you want to spice up your smoothies then natural flavoured stevia drops are amazing or a sprinkle of PB2 powder

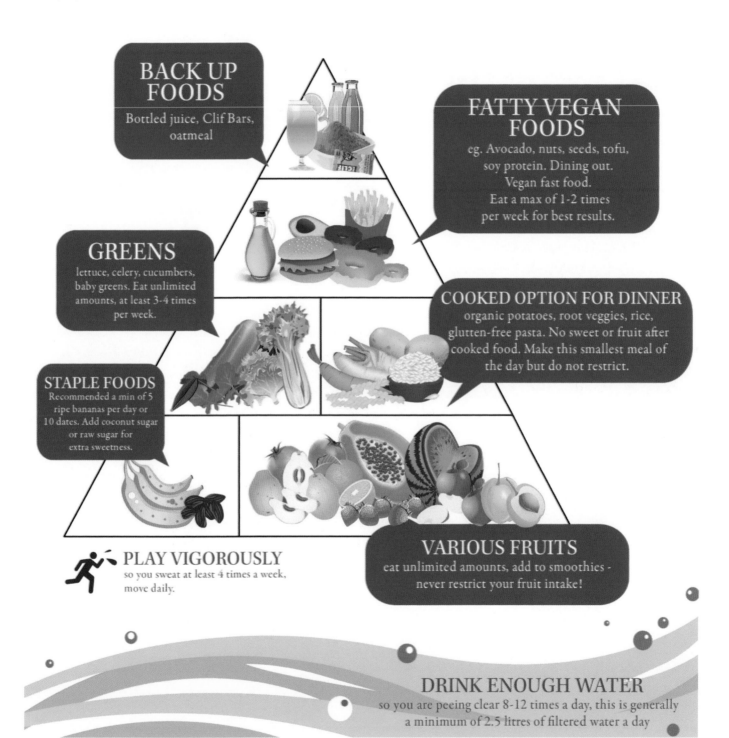

**BACK UP FOODS**
Bottled juice, Clif Bars, oatmeal

**FATTY VEGAN FOODS**
eg. Avocado, nuts, seeds, tofu, soy protein. Dining out. Vegan fast food. Eat a max of 1-2 times per week for best results.

**GREENS**
lettuce, celery, cucumbers, baby greens. Eat unlimited amounts, at least 3-4 times per week.

**COOKED OPTION FOR DINNER**
organic potatoes, root veggies, rice, glutten-free pasta. No sweet or fruit after cooked food. Make this smallest meal of the day but do not restrict.

**STAPLE FOODS**
Recommended a min of 5 ripe bananas per day or 10 dates. Add coconut sugar or raw sugar for extra sweetness.

**PLAY VIGOROUSLY**
so you sweat at least 4 times a week, move daily.

**VARIOUS FRUITS**
eat unlimited amounts, add to smoothies - never restrict your fruit intake!

**DRINK ENOUGH WATER**
so you are peeing clear 8-12 times a day, this is generally a minimum of 2.5 litres of filtered water a day

# MEALPLANNER

You made it! Now that you've educated yourself on why this lifestyle rocks, it's time to start munching your way to that happy, healthy body and mind. The calories outlined in this meal planner are of breakfast, lunch and dinner, and are not inclusive of the afternoon snack of fruit. Some people may choose to have this snack while others will not. Any foods which are classed as optional are not included in the calorie and macronutrient outlines. As you can see from the planner, carbohydrates mainly from fruit and to a lesser extent potatoes, are where the main focus of calories come from.

Remember these calorie suggestions are merely an example and are in no way a calorie or macronutrient maximum. If you want to eat more than outlined in the planner, please feel free to satisfy your hunger at every meal. This is not a calorie restriction diet and I encourage you to satiate yourself with the right types of foods. The planner was designed for females, however males are welcome to follow this guide but should take note that men generally require more calories than females and should dramatically increase their intakes, roughly by about 1000 calories. Coconut sugar is an optional addition, it improves taste and satiation and I regularly add it to my diet. If you want to substitute with other vegan sweeteners such as raw sugar, maple syrup, or date sugar then feel free to do so. This food plan strictly does not include animals products. That means no meat or seafood, no animal milk or dairy, no eggs and no honey, as this is a vegan or plant based food plan.

Remember to fill out your daily diary provided within this book to keep you on track.

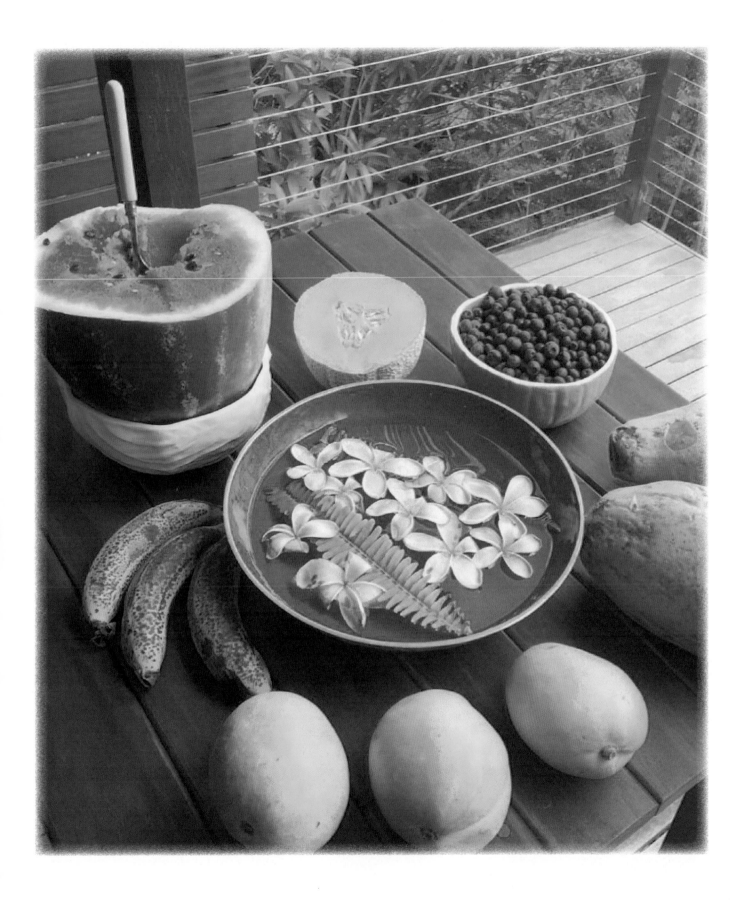

# FREELEE RECOMMENDS CALORIE STUFFING!!

There are some girls on the internet who misrepresent Raw Till 4 and my recommendations. They will say "Freelee is a calorie stuffer! She said I MUST eat 2500 calories a day or more or I fail RT4!". This is just nonsense. I have never said that. It is an excuse by these girls to quit the program and jump onto a new diet. They treat the RT4 lifestyle as a weight loss diet for the summer rather than the healing lifestyle that it is. I have only ever given recommendations as to what I have seen keep girls happy and thriving on this lifestyle. I give recommendations because I actually care! I want to see you feeling and looking your best, and after 12 years on a high fruit and RT4 lifestyle, I know what works long term. I could easily give you a starvation plan of 1600 calories like so many popular bikini body hucksters out there but again, I actually care. You are welcome to eat as much OR as little as you like but I will not recommend anything below 2100 calories for any girl, any weight, any height, as anything below 2100 calories per day is considered a famine/starvation condition by the World Health Organisation. I rally against these starvation plans, not recommend them! For this reason, you will see the calories of the meal planner sit around 2300 per day. Again this is just a recommendation, please eat MORE if you feel like it! If you feel like eating 2100 calories that day, then do that. Adjust the meal planner to suit your appetite and lifestyle desire. Without objective clear caloric recommendations, the failure rate is high because noobs to the lifestyle think that eating 1 banana for breakfast and 2 apples for lunch is enough because they 'feel' full. Feeling full is very subjective and that is why you need to listen to those thriving on this lifestyle long term. Trust me, under-eating can be a disaster for your goals and before long I see these girls going back to eating animals, feeling terrible and blaming the lifestyle for their results rather than their lack of education and commitment. So with all that said, I encourage you to eat up and enjoy yourself!

# WHEN YOU NEED A BACK UP PLAN

I understand that sometimes you just don't have any fruit available but you can ALWAYS find oats! For those times when you are stuck for fruit I recommend you buy oats as a back up plan. If I can make a delicious porridge recipe, then ANYONE can. There are so many porridge variations which you can find by looking through the #RawTill4 hashtag. You can substitute any of the meals in the planner with Oats when you are in a bind but when fresh fruit is available, they are best left for later on in the day. Below is one of my favourites.

## SWEET PEANUT BUTTER OATS
- 1 cup of instant oats
- 1/2 cup of boiling water
- 1/2 cup of apple juice (can replace with vanilla soy milk if desired)
- 1/4-1/2 cup (or more) of your choice of sugar
- 1 tbsp of PB2 (Peanut Butter) Powder (optional)

Boil 1/2 cup of water. Add apple juice and sugar to the oats. Add boiling water to the oats and stir. Take the oats to the desired consistency then add the PB2 powder on the top. Enjoy! It should be creamy, sweet, and satisfying especially on those cold winter days/nights.

# MEAL PLANNER TIPS

Please note if your smoothies/datorade recipes come out too thick don't be afraid to add a LOT more water. I generally have about 1.7 litres of water per 10-15 dates. Adapt to suit your taste. Regardless of what is written in the meal planner I recommend you eat as much leafy greens like lettuce, baby spinach and rocket as you like. One head of lettuce each day is a good amount to aim for. I expect you to fill out the blank journals every day of your 30 Day Banana Girl Cleanse. It will help keep you honest and motivated. Make sure you record 4 things you are grateful for every day, no matter how small. One of my daily motto's is "Every day above ground is a day to be grateful for". Ok, it's time to get started on your transformation!

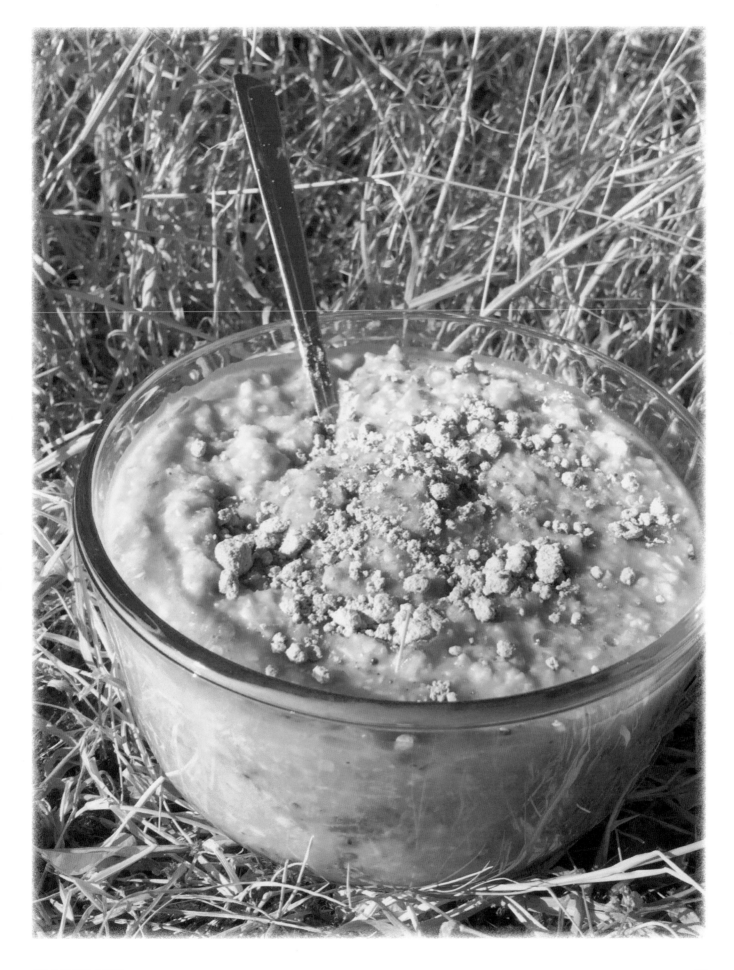

# DAY 1

## Breakfast

**Creamy RT4 Smoothie**
7 Medium Bananas
Vanilla Sweet Leaf Drops to taste
8.5 oz / 1 cup Coconut water
13 oz / 400ml Water
Optional: 1 tbsp Coconut Sugar

## Lunch

**Mono Meal of your Favourite Fruit**
4 Mangoes

## Snack

**Fruit**
Unlimited fresh fruit till 4pm

## Dinner

**#BG Fries**
500g Organic Potatoes
2 tbsp Low Sodium Dipping Sauce
1 head Lettuce
1/2 Avocado

*Calories: 2400*
*Protein: 37g - 5%*
*Carbs: 535g - 86%*
*Fat: 25g - 9%*

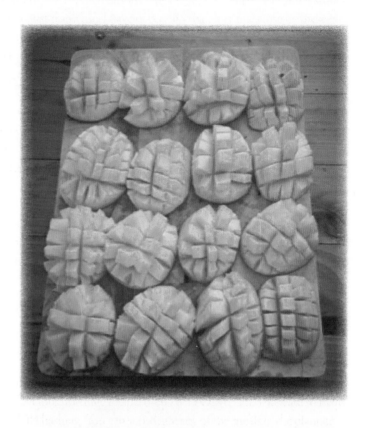

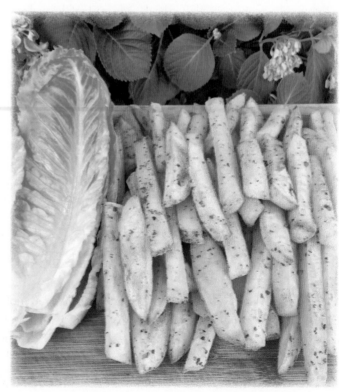

# Food Diary

| | | |
|---|---|---|
| Breakfast | | Calories: _____ |
| Lunch | | Calories: _____ |
| Dinner | | Calories: _____ |
| Snack | | Total Calories: _____ |
| Water | AM        NOON        PM | |
| Exercise | | |
| Gratitude | 1._____    2._____ <br> 3._____    4._____ | |
| Feelings | | |
| What did I do well today? | | |
| How can I improve tomorrow? | | |

**FREELEE'S TIPS:** Hydration! You want to be peeing 8-12 times per day on average and you want your urine to be clear. Aim to pee clear, if you pee and it's dark yellow or amber then you definitely need to drink more water. It's also healthy to pee once during the night.

# DAY 2

## Breakfast
**Banana Nicecream w/ Blueberry Sauce**

6 Medium Frozen Bananas
3 Medjool Dates
1/2 cup Frozen Blueberries
Optional: 1 tbsp Coconut Sugar

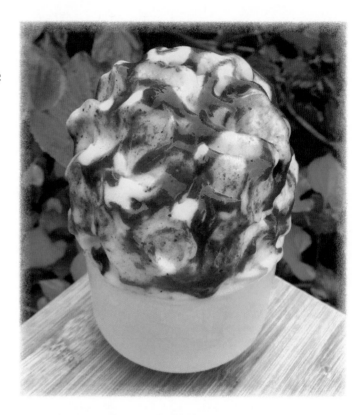

## Lunch
**Creamy Green Smoothie**

7 Medium Bananas
1 cup Baby Spinach
8.5 oz / 1 cup Non-Dairy Milk
13 oz / 400 ml Water
Optional: 1 tbsp Coconut Sugar

## Snack
**Fruit**

Unlimited fresh fruit till 4pm

## Dinner
**Pasta Napoletana**

100 grams dry Organic Corn/Rice Pasta
1/2 cup Tomato Based Pasta Sauce - Low Fat,
Low Sodium
1/2 cup canned Lentils
1 cup Mushrooms
1 head Lettuce

*Calories: 2340*
*Protein: 52g - 8%*
*Carbs: 550g - 86%*
*Fat: 16g - 6%*

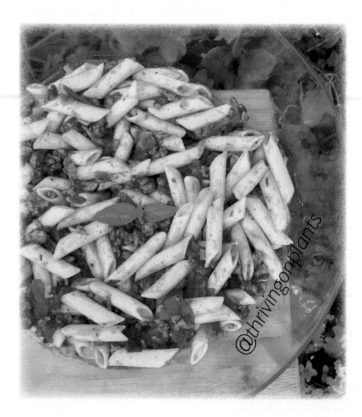

@thrivingonplants

# Food Diary

| | | |
|---|---|---|
| Breakfast | | Calories: _____ |
| Lunch | | Calories: _____ |
| Dinner | | Calories: _____ |
| Snack | | Total Calories: _____ |
| Water | AM            NOON            PM | |
| Exercise | | |
| Gratitude | 1._____  2._____  <br> 3._____  4._____ | |
| Feelings | | |
| What did I do well today? | | |
| How can I improve tomorrow? | | |

**FREELEE'S TIPS:** I recommend to drink water right after you wake up, 30 mins before big meals and during and after exercise.

# DAY 3

## Breakfast

**Datorade**

12 Medjool Dates
20 oz / 600 ml Water
Optional: 1 tbsp Coconut Sugar

## Lunch

**Mono Meal of Your Favourite Fruit**

2 Large Papayas or more

## Snack

**Fruit**

Unlimited fresh fruit till 4pm

## Dinner

**Sushi**

3/4 cup Dry Rice
Nori Sheets
1 Carrot
1 Cucumber
1 Red Pepper
1/2 Avocado

Calories: 2270
Protein: 32g - 6%
Carbs: 529g - 86%
Fat: 21g - 8%

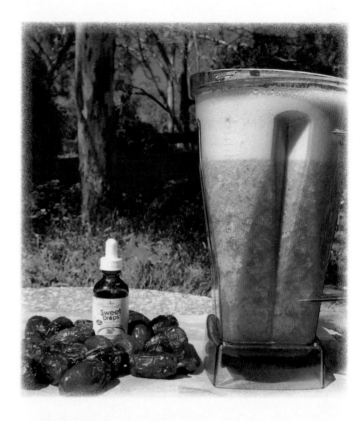

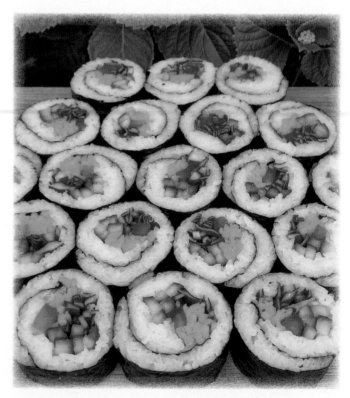

# Food Diary

| | | |
|---|---|---|
| Breakfast | | Calories: _____ |
| Lunch | | Calories: _____ |
| Dinner | | Calories: _____ |
| Snack | | Total Calories: _____ |
| Water | AM NOON PM | |
| Exercise | | |
| Gratitude | 1._____ 2._____ <br> 3._____ 4._____ | |
| Feelings | | |
| What did I do well today? | | |
| How can I improve tomorrow? | | |

**FREELEE'S TIPS:** Bananas take time to ripen, even if you have a box of ripe bananas at home, buy another box to give them time to ripen. This way you create a system where you always have ripe bananas to eat and have bananas ripening for later.

# DAY 4

## Breakfast

### #BGSNACKERS

1-2 bananas (or just dates if no bananas)
10-15 Dates
1/2 cup to 1 cup of Vanilla Soy milk
1 TBSP of PB2 choc/plain peanut powder
1.5 litres / 50 oz water
1 squirt of vanilla stevia drops (optional)

## Lunch

### Banana Nicecream w/ Carob Sauce

6 Medium Frozen Bananas
3 Medjool Dates
2 tsp Carob powder
Optional: 1 tbsp Coconut sugar

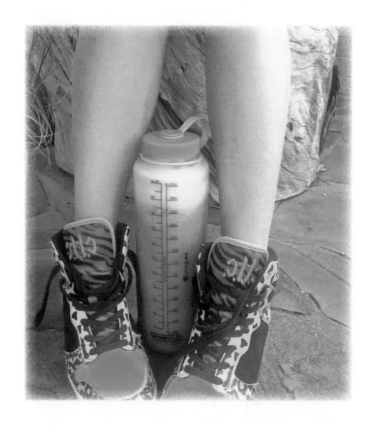

## Snack

### Fruit

Unlimited fresh fruit till 4pm

## Dinner

### Asian Style Noodles

5.3oz / 150g uncooked Rice Noodles
10.5oz / 300g Mixed Vegetables
1 tsp Sugar
1 cup / 240g / 8.5oz Vegetable Stock, or Water
2 tsp Corn Starch
1⅓ tbsp / 20g / 0.7oz Soy Sauce, Low Sodium

Calories: 2310
Protein: 42g - 6%
Carbs: 556g - 90%
Fat: 10g - 4%

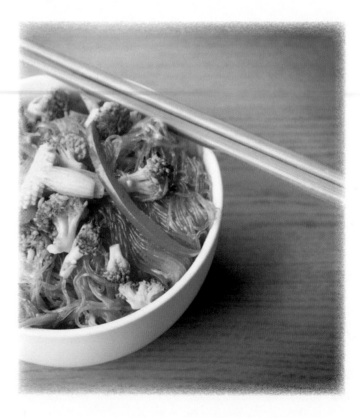

# Food Diary

| | | |
|---|---|---|
| Breakfast | | Calories: _____ |
| Lunch | | Calories: _____ |
| Dinner | | Calories: _____ |
| Snack | | Total Calories: _____ |
| Water | AM         NOON         PM | |
| Exercise | | |
| Gratitude | 1._____    2._____ <br> 3._____    4._____ | |
| Feelings | | |
| What did I do well today? | | |
| How can I improve tomorrow? | | |

**FREELEE'S TIPS:** Bananas take about a week to ripen, this totally changes depending on climate and how unripe they are. Covering them with plastic will help because it concentrates the gases they give off to make them ripen faster. Don't keep your bananas in intense heat, they will go soft and yuck .

# DAY 5

## Breakfast

**Mono Meal of Your Favourite Fruit**

22 or more Medium Fresh Figs

## Lunch

**Banana Girl Green Smoothie**

10 Medjool Dates
1 cup Frozen Strawberries
1 cup Baby Spinach
20 oz / 600 ml Water
Optional:1 tbsp Coconut Sugar

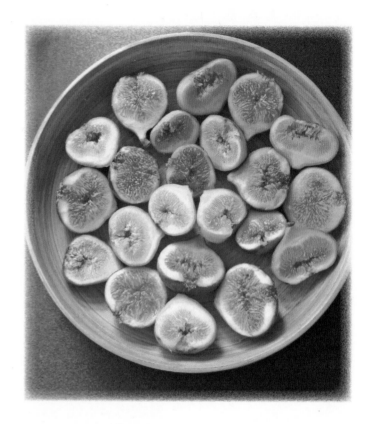

## Snack

**Fruit**

Unlimited fresh fruit till 4pm

## Dinner

**Pizza**

1.2 cup / 145g / 5.1 oz
All-Purpose /Plain Flour
1.5 tsp / 6g / 0.2oz Sugar
2/5 tsp / 1.5g / 0.05oz Instant Yeast
2/5 tsp / 2.5g / 0.1oz Salt
1 cup low sodium Pasta Sauce
1 cup raw Mushrooms
1cup Rocket / Arugula
Optional: Vegan Corner's Mozzarella Sauce
Gluten free flour can be used, just expect slightly different consistency

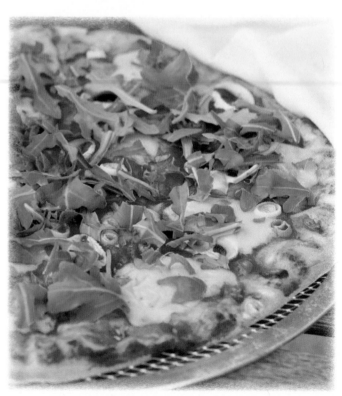

*Calories: 2250*
*Protein: 27g - 4%*
*Carbs: 554g - 92%*
*Fat: 11g - 4%*

# Food Diary

| | | |
|---|---|---|
| Breakfast | | Calories: _____ |
| Lunch | | Calories: _____ |
| Dinner | | Calories: _____ |
| Snack | | Total Calories: _____ |
| Water | AM        NOON        PM | |
| Exercise | | |
| Gratitude | 1._____    2._____ <br> 3._____    4._____ | |
| Feelings | | |
| What did I do well today? | | |
| How can I improve tomorrow? | | |

**FREELEE'S TIPS:** Cavendish bananas are ripe when they are heavily spotty. Eating them unripe i.e. not spotty, green and starchy can lead to an upset stomach and/or constipation.

# DAY 6

## Breakfast

**Apple Pie Hug**
10 Medjool Dates
1 Apple
1 tsp Warming Spice
1/2 tsp Cinnamon
20 oz / 600 ml Water
Optional:1 tbsp Coconut Sugar

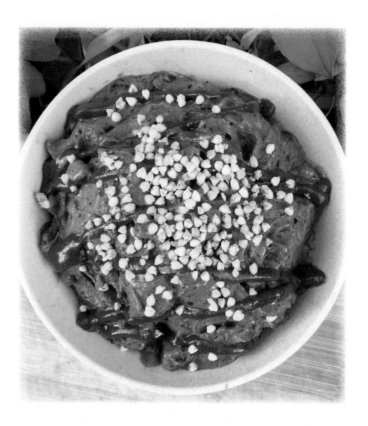

## Lunch

**Blueberry and Banana Nicecream w/ Carob  Sauce**
6 Medium Frozen Bananas
1 cup Frozen Blueberries
3 Medjool Dates
2 tsp Carob Powder
Optional: 1 tbsp Coconut Sugar and Bukinis to garnish

## Snack

**Fruit**
Unlimited fresh fruit till 4pm

## Dinner

**Dine out**
Example: Tofu with Vegetables and Rice
Ask for Vegan, Low Sodium and Low Oil

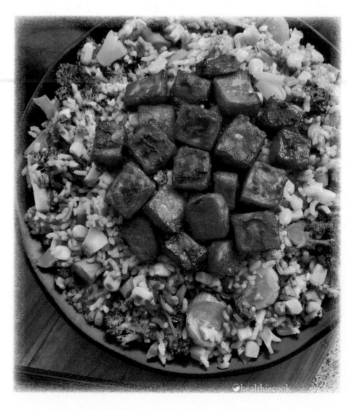

*Calories: 2560*
*Protein: 39g - 5%*
*Carbs: 566g - 82%*
*Fat: 37g - 13%*

# Food Diary

| | | |
|---|---|---|
| Breakfast | | Calories: _____ |
| Lunch | | Calories: _____ |
| Dinner | | Calories: _____ |
| Snack | | Total Calories: _____ |
| Water | AM NOON PM | |
| Exercise | | |
| Gratitude | 1._____ 2._____ 3._____ 4._____ | |
| Feelings | | |
| What did I do well today? | | |
| How can I improve tomorrow? | | |

**FREELEE'S TIPS:** Aim to keep your salt intake low and under 1000mg, under 500mg for maximum leanness. This is not an ethical issue in terms of veganism, if you choose to eat more salt, exercise will help you sweat it out of your system.

# DAY 7 #RAW24

## Breakfast

**Rockmelon Smoothie**

4 Rockmelons / Cantaloups

## Lunch

**Fresh Orange Juice**

50 oz / 1.5 L Fresh Orange Juice

## Snack

**Fruit**

More fruit!

## Dinner

**Banana Girl Apple Strudel**

4 Medium Bananas

4 Medjool Dates

1/2 cup Young Coconut Meat

1 Apple

Vanilla Sweet Leaf Drops to taste

1 tsp of Warming Spice

Optional: 1 tbsp Coconut Sugar, Cinnamon, Cardamom, Ginger, Nutmeg or Cloves Powder

*Calories: 2370*

*Protein: 38g - 5%*

*Carbs: 553g - 87%*

*Fat: 23g - 8%*

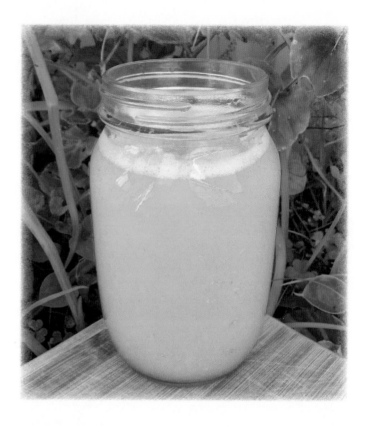

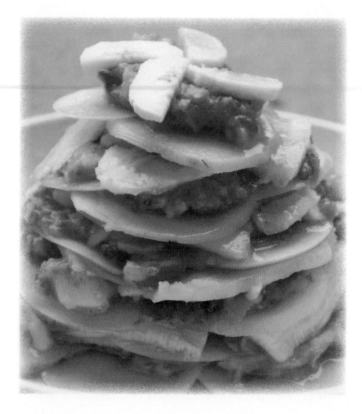

# Food Diary

| | | |
|---|---|---|
| Breakfast | | Calories: _____ |
| Lunch | | Calories: _____ |
| Dinner | | Calories: _____ |
| Snack | | Total Calories: _____ |
| Water | AM          NOON          PM | |
| Exercise | | |
| Gratitude | 1._____  2._____<br>3._____  4._____ | |
| Feelings | | |
| What did I do well today? | | |
| How can I improve tomorrow? | | |

**FREELEE'S TIPS:** Oil is not a health food, try to minimise and avoid it when possible. Oil free cooking is easy, delicious and is shown how to do in the planner.

# DAY 8

## Breakfast

**BG Berry Blast**
10 Medjool Dates
1 cup Mixed Frozen Berries
20 oz / 600 ml Water
Optional: 1 tbsp Coconut Sugar
Strain Seeds if desired.

## Lunch

**Mono Meal of Your Favourite Fruit**
Maybe 22 or more Medium Fresh Figs

## Snack

**Fruit**
Unlimited fresh fruit till 4pm

## Dinner

**Sweet Potato and Potato Fries**
250g Organic Potatoes
250g Organic Sweet Potato
Sweet Chilli Sauce - Low Sodium
1 head of Lettuce leaves
1/2 Avocado

*Calories: 2270*
*Protein: 30g - 4%*
*Carbs: 543g - 89%*
*Fat: 20g - 7%*

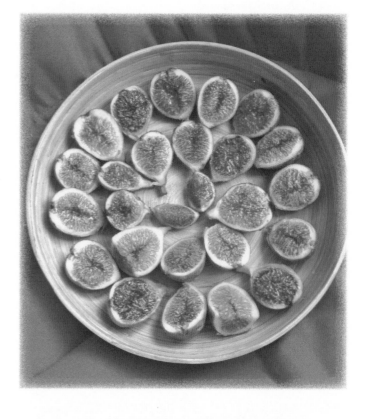

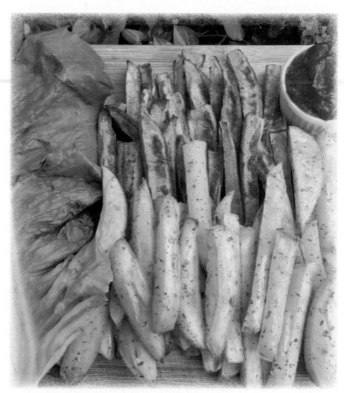

# Food Diary

| | | |
|---|---|---|
| Breakfast | | Calories: _____ |
| Lunch | | Calories: _____ |
| Dinner | | Calories: _____ |
| Snack | | Total Calories: _____ |
| Water | AM            NOON            PM | |
| Exercise | | |
| Gratitude | 1._____  2._____  3._____  4._____ | |
| Feelings | | |
| What did I do well today? | | |
| How can I improve tomorrow? | | |

**FREELEE'S TIPS:** Once you accustom to a low oil diet, you will love it because your body will get use to not having oil thicken your blood and lower its ability to get glucose into the cells. A high oil and fat diet negatively impacts the way insulin works in your body.

# DAY 9

## Breakfast

**Mixed Berry Nicecream**

6 Medium Frozen Bananas
1 cup Mixed Berries
Optional: 1 tbsp Coconut Sugar

## Lunch

**Creamy Green Smoothie**

7 Medium Bananas
1 cup Baby Spinach
8.5 oz / 1 cup Non-Dairy Milk
13 oz / 400 ml Water
Optional: 1 tbsp Coconut Sugar

## Snack

**Fruit**

Unlimited fresh fruit till 4pm

## Dinner

**Pancakes**

4.2 oz / 120 g / 1.5 cup Quick Oats
8.5 oz / 1 cup Almond Milk
1 Medium Banana
1/2 tsp Cinnamon
2-3 Medjool Dates
1-2 tbsp Carob
Optional: 1 tbsp Coconut Sugar and 3 tbsp Rice Malt Syrup

*Calories: 2300*
*Protein: 45g - 8%*
*Carbs: 536g - 84%*
*Fat: 20g - 8%*

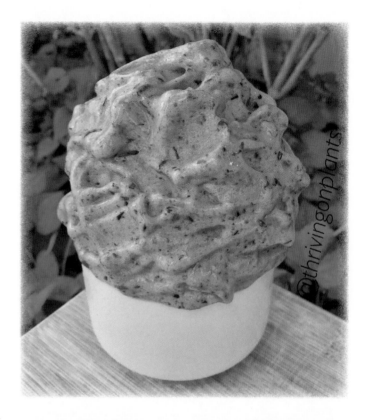

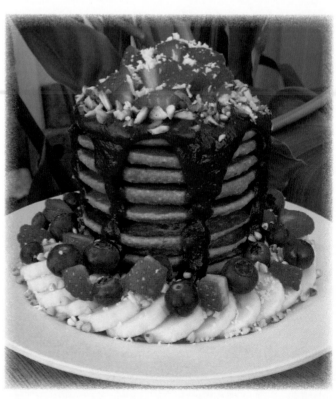

# Food Diary

| | | |
|---|---|---|
| Breakfast | | Calories: _____ |
| Lunch | | Calories: _____ |
| Dinner | | Calories: _____ |
| Snack | | Total Calories: _____ |
| Water | AM        NOON        PM | |
| Exercise | | |
| Gratitude | 1._____  2._____<br>3._____  4._____ | |
| Feelings | | |
| What did I do well today? | | |
| How can I improve tomorrow? | | |

**FREELEE'S TIPS:** Buying your staple foods in bulk and therefore at a discounted price will save you money, its a also a great idea to get to know your supplier.

# DAY 10

## Breakfast
**Mono Meal of Your Favourite Fruit**
12 Medjool Dates

## Lunch
**Meal of Your Favourite Fruit**
2 Large Papayas
1 cup Cherries

## Snack
**Fruit**
Unlimited fresh fruit till 4pm

## Dinner
**#BG Fries**
500g Organic Potatoes
Sweet Chilli Sauce - Low Sodium
1 head Lettuce leaves
1/2 Avocado

*Calories: 2292*
*Protein: 30g - 4%*
*Carbs: 547g - 88%*
*Fat: 21g - 8%*

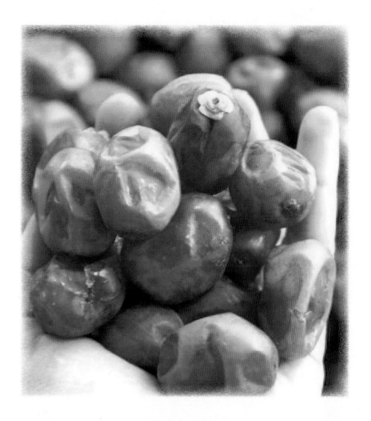

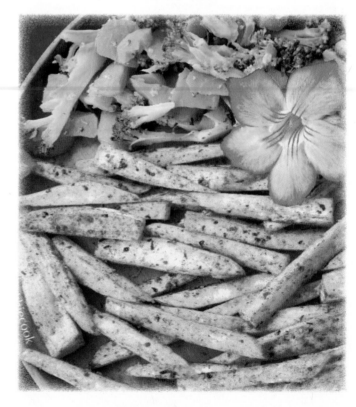

# Food Diary

| | | |
|---|---|---|
| Breakfast | | Calories: _____ |
| Lunch | | Calories: _____ |
| Dinner | | Calories: _____ |
| Snack | | Total Calories: _____ |
| Water | AM | NOON | PM |
| Exercise | | |
| Gratitude | 1._____ 2._____ <br> 3._____ 4._____ | |
| Feelings | | |
| What did I do well today? | | |
| How can I improve tomorrow? | | |

**FREELEE'S TIPS:** Always have instantly edible food on hand at home so you never have to go hungry when you're ravenousness , if that means dates, juices, crackers, frozen bananas etc something so that you don't go hungry.

# DAY 11

## Breakfast

**Banana Mango Smoothie**

5 Medium Bananas
1 Mango
8.5 oz / 1 cup Non-Dairy Milk
13 oz / 400 ml Water
Optional: 1 tbsp Coconut Sugar

## Lunch

**Papaya Nicecream with Passionfruit**

6 Medium Frozen Bananas
15 oz / 3 cups / 1/2 Large Papaya
4 Passion Fruits
Optional: 1 tbsp Coconut Sugar

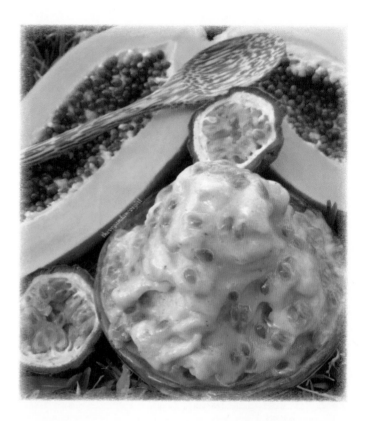

## Snack

**Fruit**

Unlimited fresh fruit till 4pm

## Dinner

**Sweet Potato Fries**

500g Organic Sweet Potatoes
Sweet Chilli Sauce - Low Sodium
1 head Lettuce leaves


*Calories: 2240*
*Protein: 42g - 6%*
*Carbs: 542g - 89%*
*Fat: 13g - 5%*

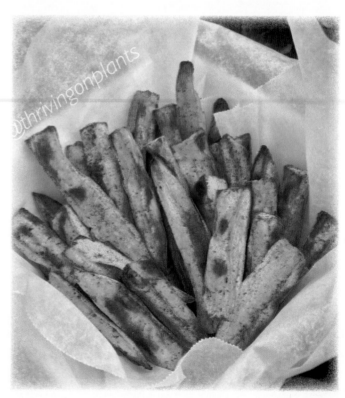

# Food Diary

| | | |
|---|---|---|
| Breakfast | | Calories: _____ |
| Lunch | | Calories: _____ |
| Dinner | | Calories: _____ |
| Snack | | Total Calories: _____ |
| Water | AM          NOON          PM | |
| Exercise | | |
| Gratitude | 1._____  2._____<br>3._____  4._____ | |
| Feelings | | |
| What did I do well today? | | |
| How can I improve tomorrow? | | |

**FREELEE'S TIPS:** Don't go out hungry. When you're out plan to have snacks in your backpack, car, gym bag etc. Being hungry when you're out and about tempts you to eat unwanted types of 'food'.

# DAY 12

## Breakfast

**Nicecream with Vanilla Date Sauce**

6 Medium Frozen Bananas
3 Medjool Dates
Vanilla Sweet Leaf Drops to taste
Optional: 1 tbsp Coconut Sugar

## Lunch

**Green Smoothie**

7 Medium Bananas
1 cup of Baby Spinach
20 oz / 600 ml Water
Optional: 1 tbsp Coconut Sugar

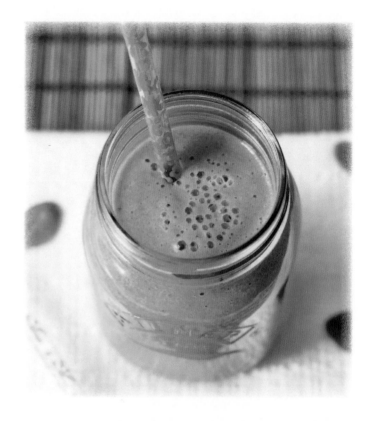

## Snack

**Fruit**

Unlimited fresh fruit till 4pm

## Dinner

**#BG Fries**

500g of Organic Potatoes
Low sodium Dipping Sauce
1 head of Lettuce
1/2 Avocado

*Calories: 2260*
*Protein: 35g - 5%*
*Carbs: 534g - 87%*
*Fat: 21g - 8%*

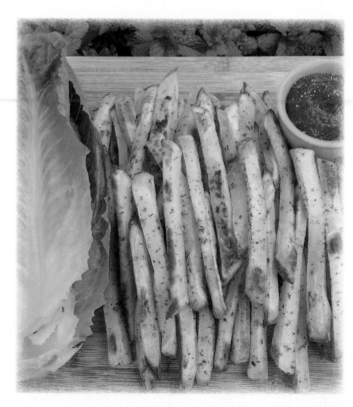

# Food Diary

| | | |
|---|---|---|
| Breakfast | | Calories: _____ |
| Lunch | | Calories: _____ |
| Dinner | | Calories: _____ |
| Snack | | Total Calories: _____ |
| Water | AM | NOON | PM |
| Exercise | | |
| Gratitude | 1._____  2._____<br>3._____  4._____ | |
| Feelings | | |
| What did I do well today? | | |
| How can I improve tomorrow? | | |

**FREELEE'S TIPS:** The number one reason people fail on the high carb vegan lifestyle is that they under eat. If you are being tempted by unwanted types of food it's a sure sign that you need to eat more.

# DAY 13

## Breakfast

**Peppermint Crisp**
12 Medjool Dates
Peppermint Sweet Leaf Drops to taste
 or Fresh Mint
20 oz / 600 ml Water
Optional: 1 tbsp Coconut Sugar

## Lunch

**Layered Berry Nicecream**
6 Medium Frozen Bananas
1/2 cup Mixed Frozen Berries
1/2 cup Frozen Strawberries
Optional: 1 tbsp Coconut Sugar

## Snack

**Fruit**
Unlimited fresh fruit till 4pm

## Dinner

**Dine out**
Example: Pizza -
Vegetables without Cheese


Calories: 2410
Protein: 28g - 6%
Carbs: 537g - 83%
Fat: 31g - 11%

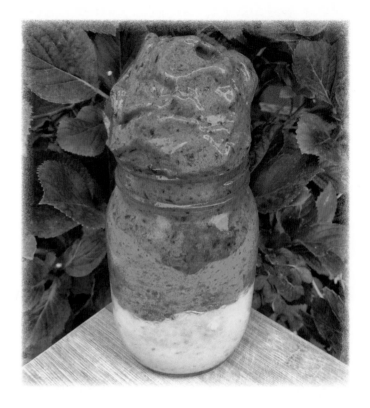

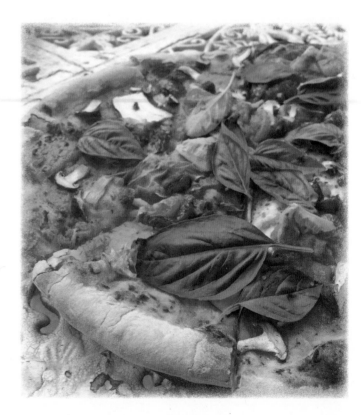

# Food Diary

| | | |
|---|---|---|
| Breakfast | | Calories: _____ |
| Lunch | | Calories: _____ |
| Dinner | | Calories: _____ |
| Snack | | Total Calories: _____ |
| Water | AM          NOON          PM | |
| Exercise | | |
| Gratitude | 1._____  2._____ <br> 3._____  4._____ | |
| Feelings | | |
| What did I do well today? | | |
| How can I improve tomorrow? | | |

**FREELEE'S TIPS:** You can substitute the baby spinach in the smoothies for other greens like celery or mixed lettuce etc, just choose your favourite greens. Also if you prefer not to have green smoothies and have the extra greens with your dinner thats fine too.

# DAY 14 #RAW24

## Breakfast
**Mono Meal of Your Favourite Fruit**
2 Large Papayas

## Lunch
**Orange Berry Smoothie**
50 oz / 1.5 L Fresh Orange Juice
1 cup Frozen Mixed Berries
Strain the seeds of desired

## Snack
**Fruit**
More fruit!

## Dinner
**Thai Mango Noodles**
4 Large Mangoes
3 Zucchinis or Cucumbers
1/2 bunch Coriander
3 sprigs Thai Basil
1 Kafir Lime Leaf
0.5 cm Lemongrass
1 lettuce head
Optional: Chilli or chilli flakes
Adjust herbs to taste

*Calories: 2410*
*Protein: 44g - 6%*
*Carbs: 596g - 89%*
*Fat: 15g - 5%*

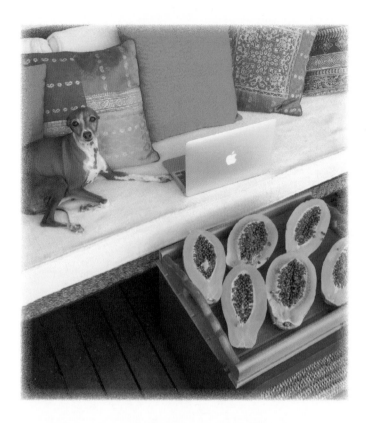

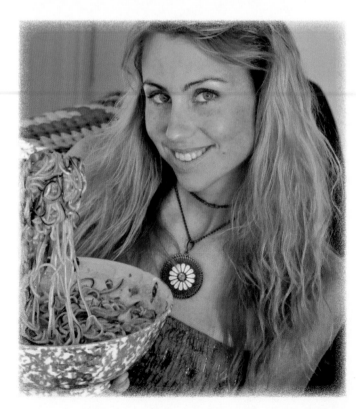

# Food Diary

| | | |
|---|---|---|
| Breakfast | | Calories: _____ |
| Lunch | | Calories: _____ |
| Dinner | | Calories: _____ |
| Snack | | Total Calories: _____ |
| Water | AM       NOON       PM | |
| Exercise | | |
| Gratitude | 1._____ 2._____ <br> 3._____ 4._____ | |
| Feelings | | |
| What did I do well today? | | |
| How can I improve tomorrow? | | |

**FREELEE'S TIPS:** You don't need to have to wait until exactly 4pm to eat cooked food. The idea is to eat raw until a couple of hours before your cooked dinner (to give the raw fruit enough time to move through your stomach). Stick to raw foods for your first two meals of the day, and try to get the majority of your calories for the day from these raw fruits.

# DAY 15

## Breakfast
**Banana Date and Coconut Water**
5 Medium Bananas
2 Medjool Dates
8.5 oz / 1 cup Coconut water
13 oz / 400ml Water
Vanilla Sweet Leaf Drops to taste
Optional: 1 tbsp Coconut Sugar

## Lunch
**Mono Meal of Your Favourite Fruit**
4 Mangoes

## Snack
**Fruit**
Unlimited fresh fruit till 4pm

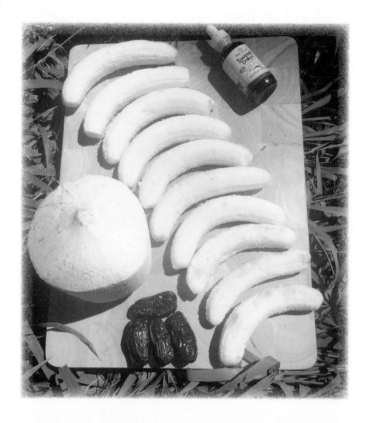

## Dinner
**#BG Fries**
500g Organic Potatoes
Sweet Chilli Sauce - Low Sodium
1 head of Lettuce
1/2 Avocado

*Calories: 2240*
*Protein: 36g - 5%*
*Carbs: 519g - 86%*
*Fat: 24g - 9%*

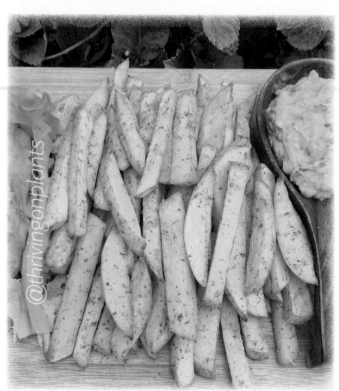

# Food Diary

| | | |
|---|---|---|
| Breakfast | | Calories: _____ |
| Lunch | | Calories: _____ |
| Dinner | | Calories: _____ |
| Snack | | Total Calories: _____ |
| Water | AM      NOON      PM | |
| Exercise | | |
| Gratitude | 1._____  2._____ <br> 3._____  4._____ | |
| Feelings | | |
| What did I do well today? | | |
| How can I improve tomorrow? | | |

**FREELEE'S TIPS:** Once you've had your cooked dinner, stay on cooked food for the rest of the day. Preferably don't eat raw fruits on top of your cooked food because the it digests much faster than the cooked starches.

# DAY 16

## Breakfast

**Banana Nicecream with Date Sauce**

6 Medium Frozen Bananas
3 Medjool Dates
2 tsp Carob Powder
Optional: 1 tbsp Coconut Sugar

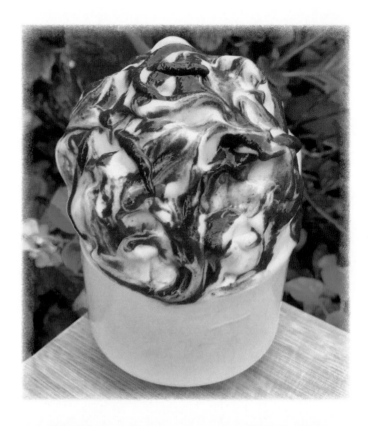

## Lunch

**Creamy Green Smoothie**

7 Medium Bananas
1 cup Baby Spinach
8.5 oz / 1 cup Non-Dairy Milk
13 oz / 400 ml Water
Optional: 1 tbsp Coconut Sugar

## Snack

**Fruit**

Unlimited fresh fruit till 4pm

## Dinner

**Sweet Potato and Potato Fries**

250g Organic Potatoes
250g Organic Sweet Potato
Sweet Chilli Sauce - Low Sodium
1 head of Lettuce Leaves

*Calories: 2240*
*Protein: 40g - 6%*
*Carbs: 544g - 90%*
*Fat: 11g - 4%*

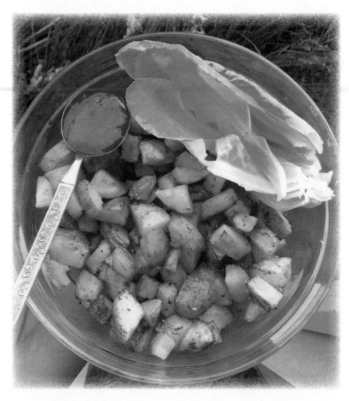

# Food Diary

| | | |
|---|---|---|
| Breakfast | | Calories: _____ |
| Lunch | | Calories: _____ |
| Dinner | | Calories: _____ |
| Snack | | Total Calories: _____ |
| Water | AM               NOON               PM | |
| Exercise | | |
| Gratitude | 1._____  2._____<br>3._____  4._____ | |
| Feelings | | |
| What did I do well today? | | |
| How can I improve tomorrow? | | |

**FREELEE'S TIPS:** There's no such thing as emotional eating. If you feel like eating then your brain and body is running low on glucose which means you need FUEL aka carbohydrates.

# DAY 17

## Breakfast

**Banana Strawberry Smoothie**

7 Medium Bananas
1 cup Strawberries
20 oz / 600ml Water
Optional: 1 tbsp Coconut Sugar

## Lunch

**Mono Meal of Your Favourite Fruit**

37 oz / 1 kg Grapes

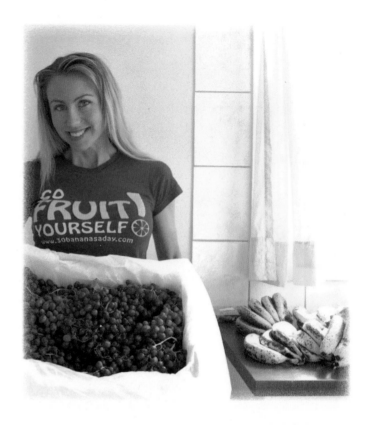

## Snack

**Fruit**
Unlimited fresh fruit till 4pm

## Dinner

**Pasta Alla Carbonara**

7oz / 200g uncooked Spaghetti
7oz / 200g / 1 Zucchini
2oz / 60g 1 Carrots, boiled
0.5oz / 15g Miso Paste
pinch of Smoked Paprika
⅛ tsp Garlic Granules
⅛ tsp Onion Granules
1 tsp / 3g All-Purpose Flour
3 tbsp / 10g / 0.3oz Nutritional Yeast
½ cup +1 tbsp/ 135g / 4.7oz non-dairy milk
1 lettuce head

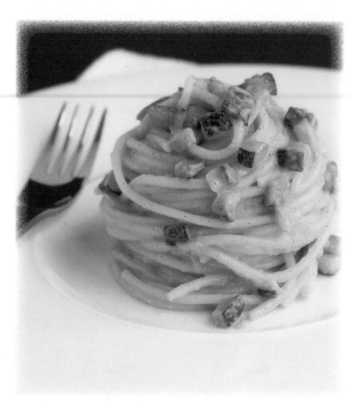

Calories: 2440
Protein: 45g - 7%
Carbs: 581g - 88%
Fat: 15g- 5%

# Food Diary

| | | |
|---|---|---|
| Breakfast | | Calories: _____ |
| Lunch | | Calories: _____ |
| Dinner | | Calories: _____ |
| Snack | | Total Calories: _____ |
| Water | AM          NOON          PM | |
| Exercise | | |
| Gratitude | 1._____  2._____<br>3._____  4._____ | |
| Feelings | | |
| What did I do well today? | | |
| How can I improve tomorrow? | | |

**FREELEE'S TIPS:** Chew your smoothies and don't guzzle them, the enzymes in your salvia will start to break down the carbohydrates and the stomach will receive the contents at a more gradual rate. Its also a good idea to rinse your mouth with water or brush your teeth afterwards for good dental care.

# DAY 18

## Breakfast

**Banana Mango Smoothie**

5 Medium Bananas
1 Mango
8 oz / 1 cup Non-Dairy Milk
13 oz / 400 ml Water
Optional: 1 tbsp Coconut Sugar

## Lunch

**Summer Smoothie Bowl**

1 Large Mango
1/2 Large Papaya
2 Passion Fruits
4 Medium Bananas
Optional: 1 tbsp Coconut Sugar

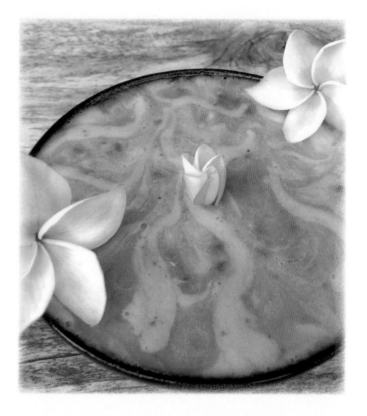

## Snack

**Fruit**
Unlimited fresh fruit till 4pm

## Dinner

**#BG Fries**

500g Organic Potatoes
Tomato Sauce - Low Sodium
1 head of Lettuce Leaves

*Calories: 2180*
*Protein: 41g - 6%*
*Carbs: 524g - 89%*
*Fat: 13g - 5%*

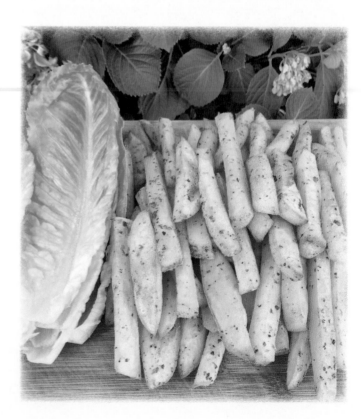

# Food Diary

| | | |
|---|---|---|
| Breakfast | | Calories: _____ |
| Lunch | | Calories: _____ |
| Dinner | | Calories: _____ |
| Snack | | Total Calories: _____ |
| Water | AM        NOON        PM | |
| Exercise | | |
| Gratitude | 1._____  2._____<br>3._____  4._____ | |
| Feelings | | |
| What did I do well today? | | |
| How can I improve tomorrow? | | |

**FREELEE'S TIPS:** How to improve any initial feelings of bloating: ensure you are combining food properly, eat slowly, be hydrated and drink water before meals, minimise your salt intake and try not to eat late at night.

# DAY 19

## Breakfast
**Vanilla Nice Cream with Blueberries**
7 Medium Frozen Bananas
Vanilla Sweet Leaf Drops to taste
1 Cup Fresh Blueberries

## Lunch
**Green Smoothie**
7 Medium Bananas
1 cup Baby Spinach
20 oz / 600 ml Water
Optional: 1 tbsp Coconut Sugar

## Snack
**Fruit**
Unlimited fresh fruit till 4pm

## Dinner
**Sweet Potato Fries**
500g Organic Sweet Potatoes
Sweet Chilli Sauce - Low Sodium
1 head of Lettuce leaves
1/2 Avocado

*Calories: 2270*
*Protein: 36g - 5%*
*Carbs: 533g - 87%*
*Fat: 23g - 8%*

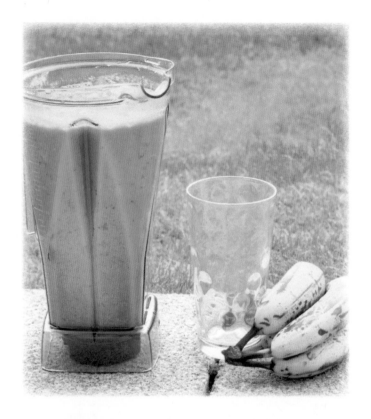
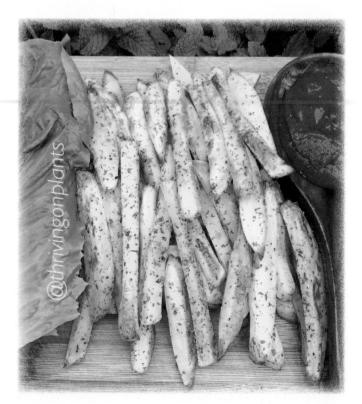

# Food Diary

| | | |
|---|---|---|
| Breakfast | | Calories: _____ |
| Lunch | | Calories: _____ |
| Dinner | | Calories: _____ |
| Snack | | Total Calories: _____ |
| Water | AM                    NOON                    PM | |
| Exercise | | |
| Gratitude | 1._____   2._____<br>3._____   4._____ | |
| Feelings | | |
| What did I do well today? | | |
| How can I improve tomorrow? | | |

**FREELEE'S TIPS:** To get the full benefits from the lifestyle you must combine proper sleep, water, food and exercise.

# DAY 20

## Breakfast

**BG Berry Blast**
10 Medjool Dates
1 Cup Mixed Frozen Berries
20 oz / 600 ml Water
Optional: 1 tbsp Coconut Sugar
Strain Seeds if Desired

## Lunch

**Nice Cream**
7 Medium Frozen Bananas
Optional: 1 tbsp Coconut Sugar

## Snack

**Fruit**
Unlimited fresh fruit till 4pm

## Dinner

**Dine out**
Example: Chickpea and Vegetable
Curry with Rice

Calories: 2600
Protein: 36g - 5%
Carbs: 555g - 80%
Fat: 43g - 15%

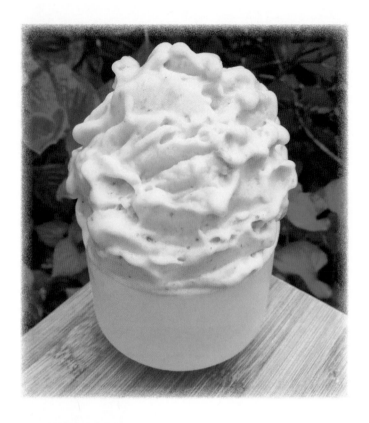

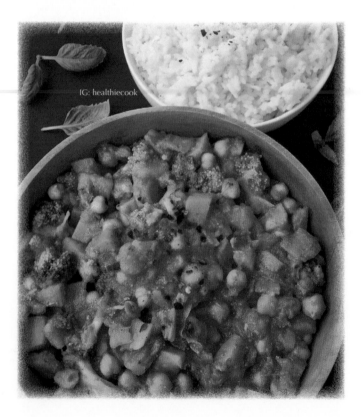

IG: healthiecook

# Food Diary

| | | |
|---|---|---|
| Breakfast | | Calories: _____ |
| Lunch | | Calories: _____ |
| Dinner | | Calories: _____ |
| Snack | | Total Calories: _____ |
| Water | AM        NOON        PM | |
| Exercise | | |
| Gratitude | 1._____ 2._____ <br> 3._____ 4._____ | |
| Feelings | | |
| What did I do well today? | | |
| How can I improve tomorrow? | | |

**FREELEE'S TIPS:** Aim to get 8-12 hours of sleep a night and try to be in bed before 9pm.

# DAY 21 #RAW24

## Breakfast

**Watermelon**

15 cups / 80 oz / 2.3kg /
half a Watermelon
(1 whole Watermelon which is approx 15inches x 7 inches /
38cm x 18cm)

## Lunch

**Mono Meal of Your Favourite Fruit**

Maybe 10 Ripe Oranges

## Snack

**Fruit**

Unlimited fresh fruit till 4pm

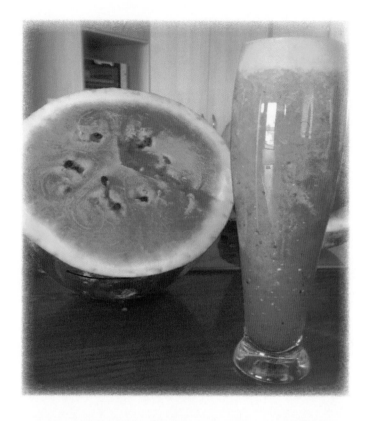

## Dinner

**Tropical Fruit Soup**

4 Medium Bananas
1 Young Coconut - the Meat and Water
1 Large Papaya
Optional: Water for Desired Consistency

Calories: 2400
Protein: 39g - 5%
Carbs: 583g - 88%
Fat: 19g - 7%

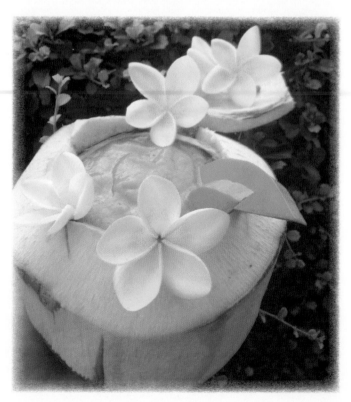

# Food Diary

| | | |
|---|---|---|
| Breakfast | | Calories: _____ |
| Lunch | | Calories: _____ |
| Dinner | | Calories: _____ |
| Snack | | Total Calories: _____ |
| Water | AM         NOON        PM | |
| Exercise | | |
| Gratitude | 1._____ 2._____<br>3._____ 4._____ | |
| Feelings | | |
| What did I do well today? | | |
| How can I improve tomorrow? | | |

**FREELEE'S TIPS:** Good health is not something we can buy, however it is priceless.

# DAY 22

## Breakfast

**Datorade**
12 Medjool Dates
20 oz / 600 ml Water
Optional: 1 tbsp Coconut Sugar

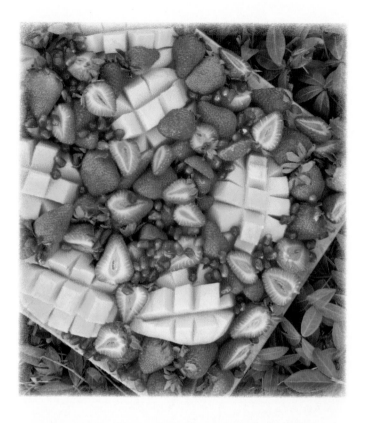

## Lunch

**Mono Meal of Your Favourite Fruit**
4 Large Mangoes
1 cup Strawberries

## Snack

**Fruit**
Unlimited fresh fruit till 4pm

## Dinner

**Sweet Potato and Potato Fries**
250g Organic Potatoes
250g Organic Sweet Potato
Dipping Sauce - Low Sodium
1 head of Lettuce leaves
1/2 Avocado

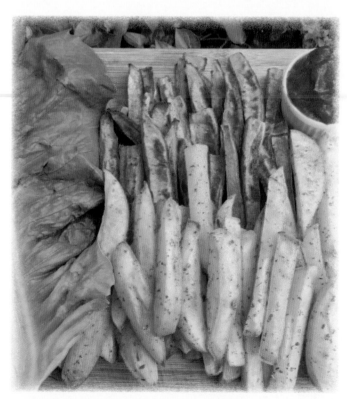

*Calories: 2240*
*Protein: 32g - 5%*
*Carbs: 517g - 87%*
*Fat: 22g - 8%*

# Food Diary

| | | | |
|---|---|---|---|
| Breakfast | | | Calories: _____ |
| Lunch | | | Calories: _____ |
| Dinner | | | Calories: _____ |
| Snack | | | Total Calories: _____ |
| Water | AM | NOON | PM |
| Exercise | | | |
| Gratitude | 1._____ 2._____<br>3._____ 4._____ | | |
| Feelings | | | |
| What did I do well today? | | | |
| How can I improve tomorrow? | | | |

**FREELEE'S TIPS:** Better health leads to a better life.

# DAY 23

## Breakfast

**Vanilla Nice Cream with Mango**

6 Medium Frozen Bananas

Vanilla Sweet Leaf Drops to taste

1 Large Mango

Optional: 1 tbsp Coconut Sugar

## Lunch

**Creamy Green Smoothie**

7 Medium Bananas

1 cup Baby Spinach

8 oz / 1 cup Non-Dairy Milk

13 oz / 400ml Water

Optional: 1 tbsp Coconut Sugar

## Snack

**Fruit**

Unlimited fresh fruit till 4pm

## Dinner

**Lebanese Pizza**

2 Lebanese Bread

1 cup Pasta Sauce - Low Sodium

1 cup Mushrooms

2 tbsp Hummus (vegan)

1 cup Baby Spinach

1 Tomato

Italian Herbs

Calories: 2360

Protein: 55g - 9%

Carbs: 537g - 84%

Fat: 18g - 7%

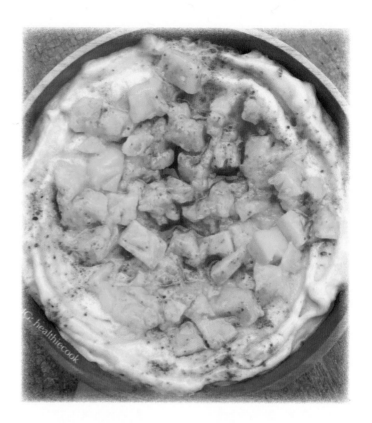

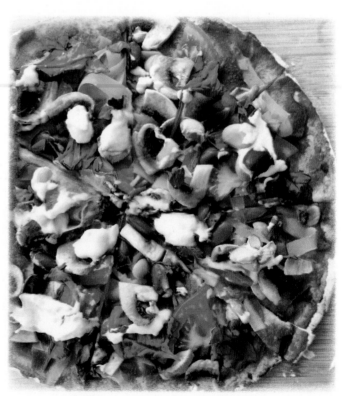

# Food Diary

| | | |
|---|---|---|
| Breakfast | | Calories: _____ |
| Lunch | | Calories: _____ |
| Dinner | | Calories: _____ |
| Snack | | Total Calories: _____ |
| Water | AM        NOON        PM | |
| Exercise | | |
| Gratitude | 1._____  2._____<br>3._____  4._____ | |
| Feelings | | |
| What did I do well today? | | |
| How can I improve tomorrow? | | |

**FREELEE'S TIPS:** Nourish your body with real food and feel it say thank you.

# DAY 24

## Breakfast

**BG Berry Blast**
10 Medjool Dates
1 Cup Mixed Frozen Berries
20 oz / 600 ml Water
Optional: 1 tbsp Coconut Sugar
Strain Seeds if Desired

## Lunch

**Mono Meal of Your Favourite Fruit**
2 Large Papayas

## Snack

**Fruit**
Unlimited fresh fruit till 4pm

## Dinner

**#BG Fries**
500g Organic Potatoes
Sweet Chilli Sauce - Low Sodium
1 head of Lettuce leaves
1/2 Avocado

*Calories: 2270*
*Protein: 30g - 4%*
*Carbs: 540g - 88%*
*Fat: 21g - 8%*

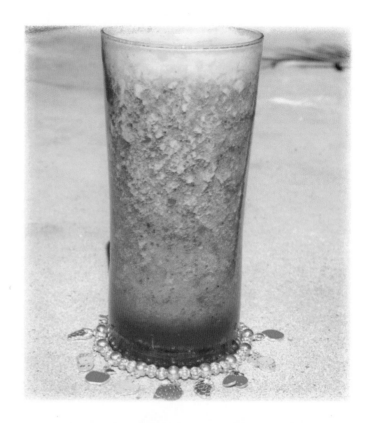

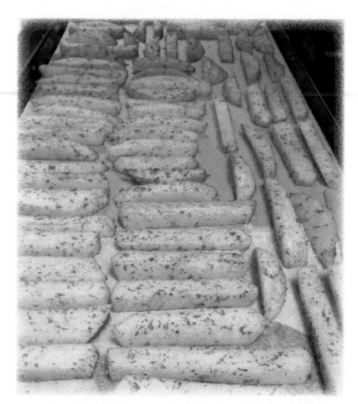

# Food Diary

| | | |
|---|---|---|
| Breakfast | | Calories: _____ |
| Lunch | | Calories: _____ |
| Dinner | | Calories: _____ |
| Snack | | Total Calories: _____ |
| Water | AM          NOON          PM | |
| Exercise | | |
| Gratitude | 1._____  2._____ <br> 3._____  4._____ | |
| Feelings | | |
| What did I do well today? | | |
| How can I improve tomorrow? | | |

**FREELEE'S TIPS:** Why pay to end the lives of innocent animals when you don't have to? This lifestyle is delicious, healthy and compassionate.

# DAY 25

## Breakfast
**Banana Mango Smoothie**
5 Medium Bananas
1 Mangoes
13 oz / 400ml Water
Optional: 1 tbsp Coconut Sugar

## Lunch
**Mango Berry Banana Nicecream**
7 Medium Frozen Bananas
1 cup Mixed Berries
1 Mango
4 Strawberries
Vanilla Sweet Leaf Drops to taste
Optional: 1 tbsp Coconut Sugar

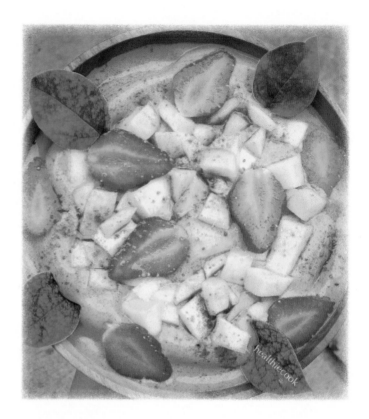

## Snack
**Fruit**
Unlimited fresh fruit till 4pm

## Dinner
**Sweet Potato Fries**
500g Organic Potatoes
Sweet Chilli Sauce - Low Sodium
1 head of Lettuce Leaves

Calories: 2310
Protein: 36g - 5%
Carbs: 574g - 92%
Fat: 9g - 3%

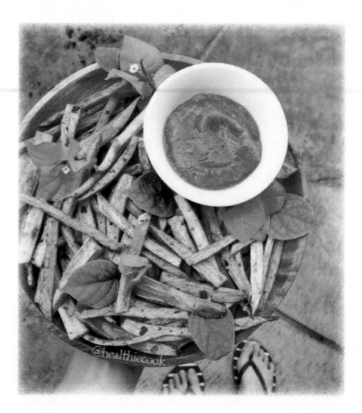

# Food Diary

| | | |
|---|---|---|
| Breakfast | | Calories: _____ |
| Lunch | | Calories: _____ |
| Dinner | | Calories: _____ |
| Snack | | Total Calories: _____ |
| Water | AM           NOON         PM | |
| Exercise | | |
| Gratitude | 1._____ 2._____ <br> 3._____ 4._____ | |
| Feelings | | |
| What did I do well today? | | |
| How can I improve tomorrow? | | |

**FREELEE'S TIPS:** No more calorie restricting or going hungry again. This lifestyle is about abundance at every meal, so that you feel satisfied and have the energy to live to the fullest.

# DAY 26

## Breakfast

**Mango Passionfruit Banana Parfait**

4 Medium Frozen Bananas
2 Mangoes
3 Passion Fruits
Optional: 1 tbsp Coconut Sugar

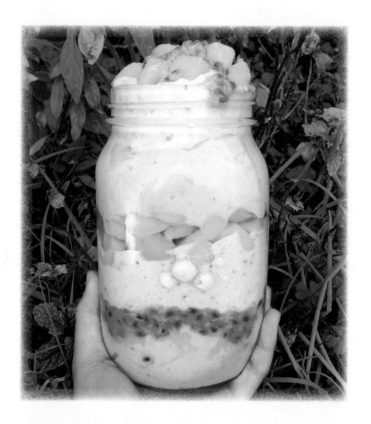

## Lunch

**Banana Girl Green Smoothie**

10 Medjool Dates
1 cup Frozen Strawberries
1 cup Baby Spinach
20 oz / 600 ml Water
Optional: 1 tbsp Coconut Sugar

## Snack

**Fruit**

Unlimited fresh fruit till 4pm

## Dinner

**#BG Fries**

500g of Organic Potatoes
Low sodium Dipping Sauce
1 head of Lettuce
1/2 Avocado

*Calories: 2310*
*Protein: 36g - 5%*
*Carbs: 548g - 87%*
*Fat: 21g - 8%*

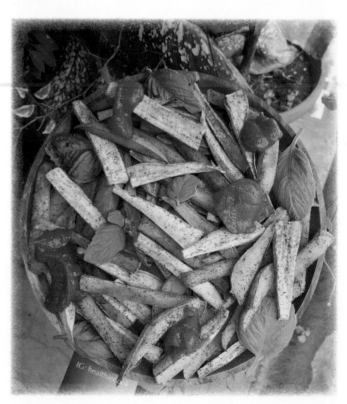

# Food Diary

| | | |
|---|---|---|
| Breakfast | | Calories: _____ |
| Lunch | | Calories: _____ |
| Dinner | | Calories: _____ |
| Snack | | Total Calories: _____ |
| Water | AM | NOON | PM |
| Exercise | | |
| Gratitude | 1._____  2._____ <br> 3._____  4._____ | |
| Feelings | | |
| What did I do well today? | | |
| How can I improve tomorrow? | | |

**FREELEE'S TIPS:** In 30 days you can learn how to re-gain your health, what have you got to lose?

# DAY 27

## Breakfast

**Mixed Berry Banana Nicecream**
7 Medium Frozen Bananas
1 cup Mixed Berries
Optional: 1 tbsp Coconut Sugar

## Lunch

**Meal of Your Favourite Fruit**
15 Figs
1 cup Blueberries
1 cup Blackberries
1cup Strawberries

## Snack

**Fruit**
Unlimited fresh fruit till 4pm

## Dinner

**Dine out - Sushi**
Example - Sushi
Mushroom, Cucumber, Tofu, Avocado

Calories: 2520
Protein: 53g - 8%
Carbs: 539g - 79%
Fat: 37g - 13%

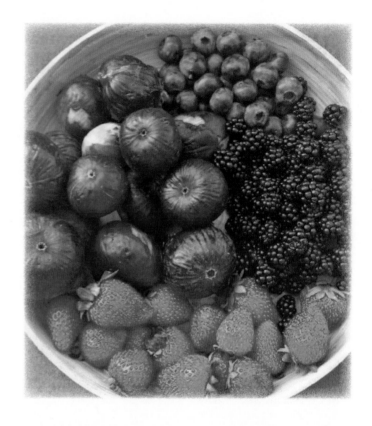

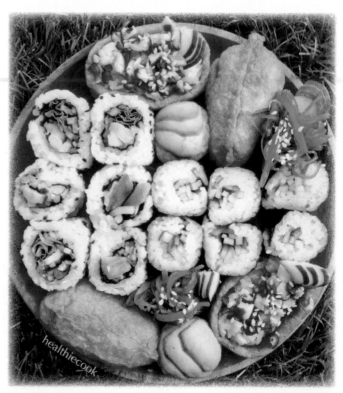

# Food Diary

| | | |
|---|---|---|
| Breakfast | | Calories: _____ |
| Lunch | | Calories: _____ |
| Dinner | | Calories: _____ |
| Snack | | Total Calories: _____ |
| Water | AM        NOON        PM | |
| Exercise | | |
| Gratitude | 1._____  2._____<br>3._____  4._____ | |
| Feelings | | |
| What did I do well today? | | |
| How can I improve tomorrow? | | |

**FREELEE'S TIPS:** It is important to eat until you are satisfied. Never eat less because you want to lose weight, this will lead to failure on the lifestyle.

# DAY 28 #RAW24

## Breakfast

**Mono Meal of Your Favourite Fruit**

37 oz / 1 kg / 7 cups Grapes

## Lunch

**Meal of your Favourite Fruit**

10 or more ripe Oranges

## Snack

**Fruit**

More Fruit!

## Dinner

**Mixed Berries and Chia Nicecream**

6 Medium Frozen Bananas

1 cup Mixed Berries

4 tbsp Chia Seeds

Optional: 1 tbsp Coconut Sugar, Strawberries and Pomegranates

*Calories: 2310*

*Protein: 36g - 5%*

*Carbs: 562g - 88%*

*Fat: 18g - 7%*

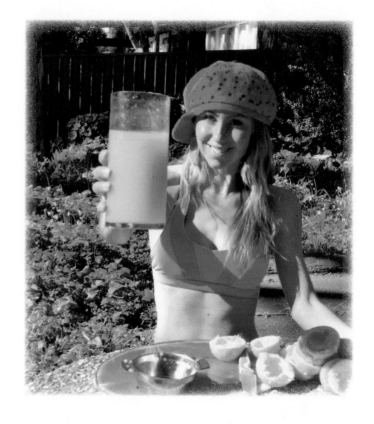

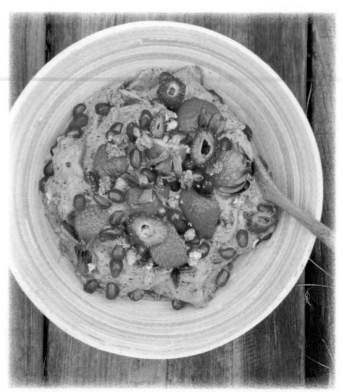

# Food Diary

| | | |
|---|---|---|
| Breakfast | | Calories: _____ |
| Lunch | | Calories: _____ |
| Dinner | | Calories: _____ |
| Snack | | Total Calories: _____ |
| Water | AM          NOON          PM | |
| Exercise | | |
| Gratitude | 1._____  2._____<br>3._____  4._____ | |
| Feelings | | |
| What did I do well today? | | |
| How can I improve tomorrow? | | |

**FREELEE'S TIPS:** Taking care of yourself makes you stronger for everyone in your life ... including you.

# DAY 29

## Breakfast

**Carob Banana Smoothie**

7 Medium Bananas
2 tsp Carob Powder
20 oz / 600 ml Water
Optional: 1 tbsp Coconut Sugar

## Lunch

**Mono Meal of Your Favourite Fruit**

15 Medium Peaches

## Snack

**Fruit**

Unlimited fresh fruit till 4pm

## Dinner

**Baked Potatoes**

500g Organic Potatoes
Italian Herbs, dried
Low Sodium Dipping Sauce
1 head Lettuce

Calories: 2210
Protein: 46g - 7%
Carbs: 534g - 88%
Fat: 14g - 5%

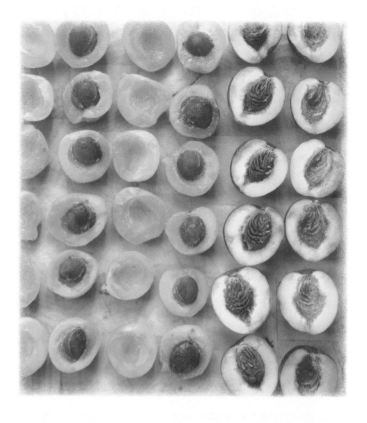

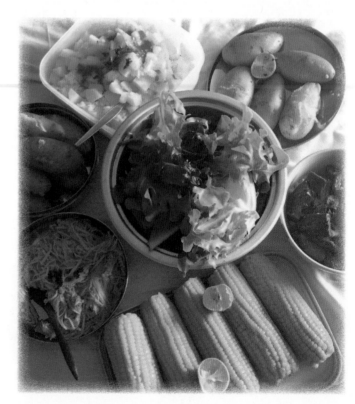

# Food Diary

| | | |
|---|---|---|
| Breakfast | | Calories: _____ |
| Lunch | | Calories: _____ |
| Dinner | | Calories: _____ |
| Snack | | Total Calories: _____ |
| Water | AM          NOON          PM | |
| Exercise | | |
| Gratitude | 1._____  2._____<br>3._____  4._____ | |
| Feelings | | |
| What did I do well today? | | |
| How can I improve tomorrow? | | |

**FREELEE'S TIPS:** Always remember you are braver than you believe, stronger than you seem, smarter than you think and twice as beautiful as you've ever imagined.

# DAY 30

## Breakfast

**Meal of your Favourite Fruit**
10 Medium Figs
4 cups / 21 oz / 600g Grapes

## Lunch

**Choc Mint Milkshake:**
12 dates
2 tsp Carob Powder
Peppermint Sweet Leaf Drops to taste
20 oz / 600ml Water
Optional: 1 tbsp Coconut Sugar

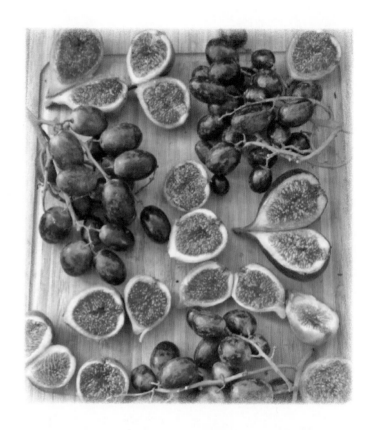

## Snack

**Fruit**
Unlimited fresh fruit till 4pm

## Dinner

**#BG Fries**
500g Organic Potatoes
Low Sodium Dipping Sauce
1 head Lettuce
1/2 Avocado

*Calories: 2370*
*Protein: 30g - 4%*
*Carbs: 574g - 89%*
*Fat: 19g - 7%*

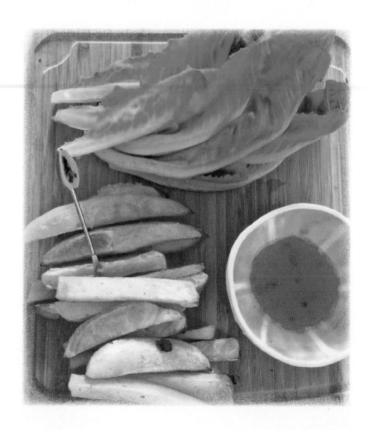

# Food Diary

| | | |
|---|---|---|
| Breakfast | | Calories: _____ |
| Lunch | | Calories: _____ |
| Dinner | | Calories: _____ |
| Snack | | Total Calories: _____ |
| Water | AM                    NOON                    PM | |
| Exercise | | |
| Gratitude | 1._____   2._____ <br> 3._____   4._____ | |
| Feelings | | |
| What did I do well today? | | |
| How can I improve tomorrow? | | |

**FREELEE'S TIPS:** If you do what you always did, you will get what you always got. It's not who you are that holds you back, it's who you think you're not.

# MACRONUTRIENT AND CALORIE AVERAGES
# FOR MEAL PLANNER

|  | Week 1 | Week 2 | Week 3 | Week 4 | Week 5 | Average of the Averages |
|---|---|---|---|---|---|---|
| **Average Total Calories** | 2357 | 2313 | 2339 | 2331 | 2290 | 2326 |
| **Average Total Protein (g)** | 38 | 36 | 39 | 40 | 38 | 38 |
| **Average Total Carbohydrate (g)** | 549 | 548 | 548 | 545 | 555 | 549 |
| **Average Total Fat (g)** | 20 | 20 | 21 | 21 | 17 | 20 |
| **Average % Protein** | 6 | 6 | 6 | 6 | 6 | 6 |
| **Average % Carbohydrate** | 87 | 87 | 87 | 86 | 88 | 87 |
| **Average % Fat** | 7 | 7 | 8 | 8 | 6 | 7 |

# ABOUT THE FRUITS INCLUDED IN
# THE MEAL PLANNER

| Fruit | Quantity | Weight Per Fruit | Weight to Make a Meal | Meal in Cals | Size in Book | Preparation |
|---|---|---|---|---|---|---|
| **Bananas** | 7 | 4.2 oz / 118 g | 29 oz / 830 g | 740 cals | Medium | Peeled |
| **Papaya** | 2 | 28 oz / 780 g | 55 oz / 1.6 kg | 670 cas | Large | Peeled and deseeded |
| **Mango** | 4 | 11.9 oz / 336 g | 47 oz / 1.3 kg | 800 cals | Large | Peeled fruit without the seed |
| **Oranges** | 10 | 4.9 oz / 140 g | 49 oz / 1.4 kg | 690 cals | Medium | Peeded |
| **Orange Juice, Fresh** | 15-20 | 5 oz / 140 g | 50 oz / 1.5 L | 700 cals | Medium | Peeled and juiced |
| **Watermelon** | 1/2 | 159.4 oz / 4518 g Measurment: Half of a 15" x 7-1/2" dia | 80 oz / 2.3 kg | 680 cals | Half a Medium | Without the rind |
| **Medjool Dates** | 12 | 0.9 oz / 24 g | 10 oz / 290 g | 800 cals | Medium | De-seeded |

# SHOPPING LIST *week 1*

## Fruit
- ☐ 22 Medium Fresh Figs
- ☐ 42 Medium Bananas (freeze 18)
- ☐ 4 Large Mangoes
- ☐ 45 Medjool Dates
- ☐ 4 Rockmelons / Cantaloups
- ☐ 1 cup Frozen Strawberries
- ☐ 1.5 cup Frozen Blueberries
- ☐ 50 oz / 1.5 L Fresh Orange Juice
- ☐ 1/2 cup Young Coconut Meat
- ☐ 2 Apples
- ☐ 2 Large Papayas

## Vegetables
- ☐ 500g of Organic Potatoes
- ☐ 5 Head Lettuce
- ☐ 1 Avocado
- ☐ 1 Cucumber
- ☐ 1 Red Pepper
- ☐ 10.5oz / 300g Mixed Vegetables
- ☐ 2 cup Baby Spinach
- ☐ 1 cup Mushrooms, raw
- ☐ 1 Carrot
- ☐ 1 cup Mushrooms, raw
- ☐ 1 cup Rocket / Arugula

## Dine Out
On Saturday night, if you choose not to dine out and prefer to cook, you could make Spicy Asian Fire Roasted Tofu if you like, here are the ingredients:

- ☐ 1/2 of a 14-16 oz block of firm tofu
- ☐ 1 heaped tbsp Asian hot sauce (Recommend Gochujang or Sriracha)
- ☐ 1 tbsp maple/coconut syrup/ coconut sugar
- ☐ 1 tbsp tomato paste
- ☐ 1 tsp soy sauce/tamari/less sodium
- ☐ Optional: 1/4 tsp white pepper powder
- ☐ Optional: 1/4 tsp black pepper powder
- ☐ Optional: 1/4 tsp garlic powder (or grate in 1 small clove)
- ☐ 200g of vegetables such as broccoli, bok choy, mushrooms etc
- ☐ 1 cup dry rice

## Vegan Corner's Mozzarella:

- [ ] 0.7oz tofu - 20g
- [ ] 0.5 cup Non-Dairy Milk - 120g / 4.3oz
- [ ] 1 tbsp + 1 tsp tapioca starch - 10g/0.4oz
- [ ] Optional: 1/4 tsp salt - 1.5g
- [ ] Optional: 1/2 small clove of garlic - 1.5g

## Optional

- [ ] 10 Tbsp Coconut Sugar
- [ ] Cinnamon, Cardamom, Ginger, Nutmeg, Cloves Powder

- [ ] Bukinis to garnish

## Shelf Item

- [ ] Vanilla Sweet Leaf Drops
- [ ] 8.5 oz / 1 cup Coconut water
- [ ] 2 tbsp Low Sodium Dipping Sauce
- [ ] 17 oz / 2 cups Non-Dairy Milk
- [ ] 100 grams dry of Organic Corn/Rice Pasta - Gluten Free
- [ ] 1/2 cup Tomato Based Pasta Sauce -
- [ ] Low Fat, Low Sodium
- [ ] 1/2 cup canned Lentils
- [ ] 3/4 cup Dry Rice
- [ ] 4 Nori Sheets
- [ ] 4 tsp Carob Powder
- [ ] 1/2 tsp cardamon powder
- [ ] 1 tsp cinnamon
- [ ] 1 cup / 240g / 8.5oz Vegetable Stock
- [ ] 2 tsp Corn Starch
- [ ] 1 tsp of Warming Spice
- [ ] 1⅓ tbsp / 20g / 0.7oz Soy Sauce, Low Sodium
- [ ] 5.3oz / 150g uncooked Rice Noodles
- [ ] 1 tsp warming spice
- [ ] 1.2 cup / 145g / 5.1 oz
- [ ] All-Purpose / Plain or Gluten Free Flour
- [ ] 2.5 tsp Sugar
- [ ] 2/5 tsp / 1.5g / 0.05oz Instant Yeast
- [ ] 2/5 tsp / 2.5g / 0.1oz Salt
- [ ] 1 cup Pasta Sauce - either use The Vegan Corner's Pizza Sauce or a store bought Low Fat, Low Sodium Pasta / Pizza Sauce

# SHOPPING LIST *week 2*

## Fruit
- ☐ 40 Medjool Dates
- ☐ 4 cup Frozen Berries
- ☐ 22 Medium Fresh Figs
- ☐ 44 Medium Bananas (freeze 24)
- ☐ 4.5 Large Papayas
- ☐ 1 cup cherries
- ☐ 4 Passion Fruits
- ☐ Peppermint Sweet Leaf Drops or Fresh Mint
- ☐ 50 oz / 1.5 L Fresh Orange Juice
- ☐ (15-20 Oranges)
- ☐ 5 Large Mangoes

## Vegetables
- ☐ 1.25 kg Organic Potatoes
- ☐ 750g Organic Sweet Potato
- ☐ 5 Head of Lettuce
- ☐ 1.5 Avocado
- ☐ 2 cup Baby Spinach
- ☐ 3 Zucchinis or Cucumbers
- ☐ 1/2 bunch Coriander
- ☐ 3 sprigs Thai Basil
- ☐ 1 Kafir Lime Leaf
- ☐ 0.5 cm Lemongrass

## Dine Out
On Saturday night, if you choose not to dine out and prefer to cook, you could make Pizza if you like, here are the ingredients:

- ☐ 1.2 cup / 145g / 5.1 oz
- ☐ All-Purpose / Plain Flour
- ☐ 1.5 tsp / 6g / 0.2oz Sugar
- ☐ 2/5 tsp / 1.5g / 0.05oz Instant Yeast
- ☐ 2/5 tsp / 2.5g / 0.1oz Salt
- ☐ 1 cup Pasta Sauce - either use The Vegan Corner's Pizza Sauce or a store bought Low Fat, Low Sodium Pasta / Pizza Sauce
- ☐ 1 cups raw Mushrooms
- ☐ 1cups Rocket / Arugula

## Vegan Corner's Mozzarella:

- ☐ 0.7oz tofu - 20g
- ☐ 0.5 cup Non-Dairy Milk - 120g / 4.3oz
- ☐ 1 tbsp + 1 tsp tapioca starch - 10g/0.4oz
- ☐ Optional: 1/4 tsp salt - 1.5g
- ☐ Optional: 1/2 small clove of garlic - 1.5g

## Optional

- ☐ 10 Tbsp Coconut Sugar
- ☐ Sweet Chilli Sauce - Low Sodium
- ☐ 3 Tbsp Rice Malt Syrup
- ☐ Chilli or chilli flakes

## Shelf Item

- ☐ 17 oz / 2 cup Non-Dairy Milk
- ☐ 4.2 oz / 120 g / 1.5 cup Quick Oats
- ☐ 8.5 oz / 1 cup Non-Dairy Milk
- ☐ Low Sodium Dipping Sauce e.g. Sweet Chilli Sauce
- ☐ 1/2 tsp Cinnamon
- ☐ 1-2 tbsp Carob
- ☐ Vanilla Sweet Leaf Drops

Note: the serving sizes for this pizza and mozzarella are half of that in the recipe section, because the ones in the recipe section give two servings. Of course if you want to eat more go ahead.

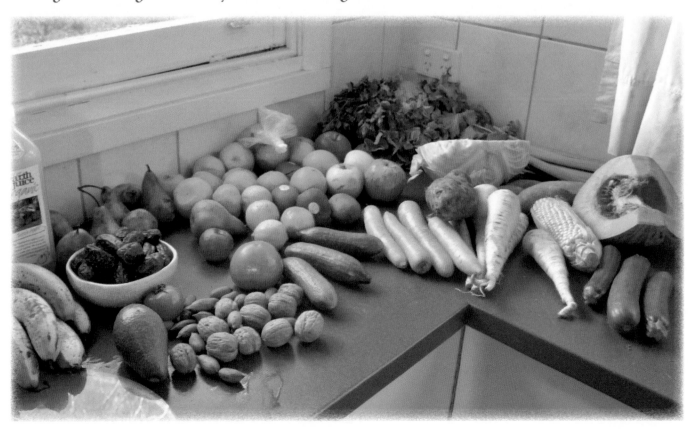

# SHOPPING LIST *week 3*

## Fruit
- [ ] 59 Medium Bananas (freeze 20)
- [ ] 15 Medjool Dates
- [ ] 8.5 oz / 1 cup Coconut water
- [ ] 1 Young Coconut - the Meat and Water
- [ ] 6 Mangoes
- [ ] 1 cup Strawberries
- [ ] 37 oz / 1 kg Grapes
- [ ] 2 Passion Fruits
- [ ] 1 Cup Blueberries, fresh
- [ ] 1 Cup Mixed Frozen Berries
- [ ] 10 Ripe Oranges
- [ ] 1.5 Large Papaya
- [ ] 15 cups / 80 oz / 2.3kg / Watermelon,
- [ ] half a watermelon where a whole watermelon is approx 15inches x 7 inches / 38cm x 18cm)

## Vegetables
- [ ] 1 cup Baby Spinach
- [ ] 1.25 kg Organic Potatoes
- [ ] 750g Organic Sweet Potato
- [ ] 5 Head of Lettuce Leaves
- [ ] 1 Avocado
- [ ] 7oz / 200g / 1 Zucchini
- [ ] 2oz / 60g 1 Carrots, boiled
- [ ] 1 cup Baby Spinach

## Dine Out
On Saturday night, if you choose not to dine out and prefer to cook, you could make Potato and Chickpea Curry if you like, here are the ingredients:

- [ ] 2 medium potatoes, peeled & chopped
- [ ] 1 (about 15oz / 400 grams) can of chickpeas, drained & rinsed
- [ ] 1 cup vegetables (I used broccoli & carrots), chopped
- [ ] 2 cloves garlic, finely chopped
- [ ] 1/2 medium onion, finely chopped
- [ ] 1 tbsp curry powder
- [ ] 1/2 tsp smoked paprika powder
- [ ] black pepper & chilli powder, to taste
- [ ] 1 tbsp coconut sugar
- [ ] 1/4 cup coconut milk

- ☐ 1/4 cup tomato paste
- ☐ water/vegetable stock, as needed
- ☐ 1 cup dry rice, cook according to package instructions, to serve

## Optional
- ☐ 8 Tbsp Coconut Sugar

## Shelf Item
- ☐ Low Sodium Dipping Sauce e.g. Sweet Chilli Sauce
- ☐ 2.5 cup Non Dairy Milk
- ☐ 2 tsp Carob Powder
- ☐ ⅛ tsp Onion Granules
- ☐ 1 tsp / 3g All-Purpose Flour
- ☐ 3 tbsp / 10g / 0.3oz Nutritional Yeast
- ☐ 7oz / 200g uncooked Spaghetti
- ☐ 0.5oz / 15g Miso Paste
- ☐ pinch of Smoked Paprika
- ☐ ⅛ tsp Garlic Granules
- ☐ Tomato Sauce - Low Sodium
- ☐ Vanilla Sweet Leaf Drops

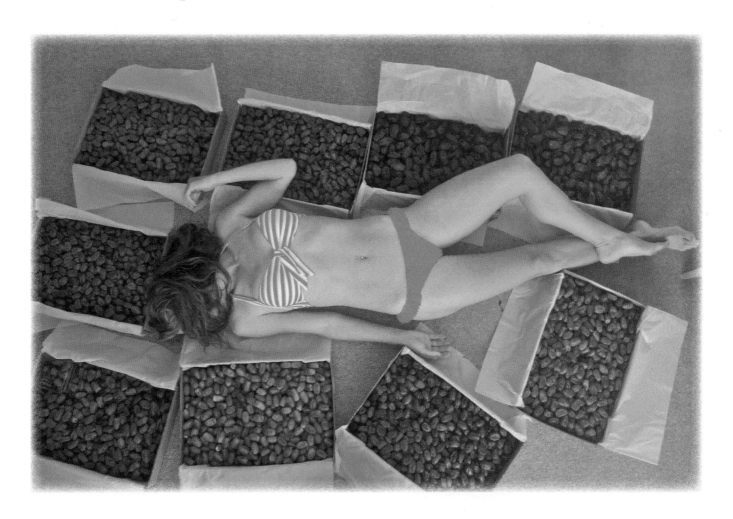

# SHOPPING LIST *week 4*

## Fruit
- [ ] 9 Large Mangoes
- [ ] 1 cup Strawberries
- [ ] 1 cup Frozen Strawberries
- [ ] 1.5 cup Strawberries, fresh
- [ ] 38 Bananas (freeze 24)
- [ ] 32 Medjool Dates
- [ ] 4 cup Mixed Frozen Berries
- [ ] 3 Passion Fruits
- [ ] 15 Figs
- [ ] 1 cup Blueberries, fresh
- [ ] 1 cup Blackberries, fresh
- [ ] 2 Large Papayas
- [ ] 37 oz / 1 kg / 7 cups Grapes
- [ ] 10 or more ripe Oranges

## Vegetables
- [ ] 3 cup Baby Spinach
- [ ] 1 cup Mushrooms
- [ ] 1 Tomato
- [ ] 1.5kg Organic Potatoes
- [ ] 1 Avocado
- [ ] 5 Head of Lettuce

## Dine Out
On Saturday night, if you choose not to dine out and prefer to cook, you could make for example Sushi, here are the ingredients:

- [ ] 3/4 cup Dry Rice
- [ ] Nori Rolls
- [ ] 0.5 Mushrooms, raw (cook for recipe)
- [ ] 1 small Cucumber
- [ ] 1/2 Avocado
- [ ] 100g Tofu
- [ ] Dipping Sauce e.g. Sweet Chilli Sauce

## Optional
- [ ] 10 Tbsp Coconut sugar
- [ ] Strawberries and Pomegranates

## Shelf Item

- [ ] 8 oz / 1 cup Non-Dairy Milk
- [ ] Vanilla Sweet Leaf Drops
- [ ] 2 Lebanese Bread
- [ ] 1 cup Pasta Sauce - Low Sodium
- [ ] 2 tbsp Hummus (vegan)
- [ ] Italian Herbs, dried or fresh
- [ ] Sweet Chilli Sauce - Low Sodium
- [ ] 4 tbsp Chia Seeds

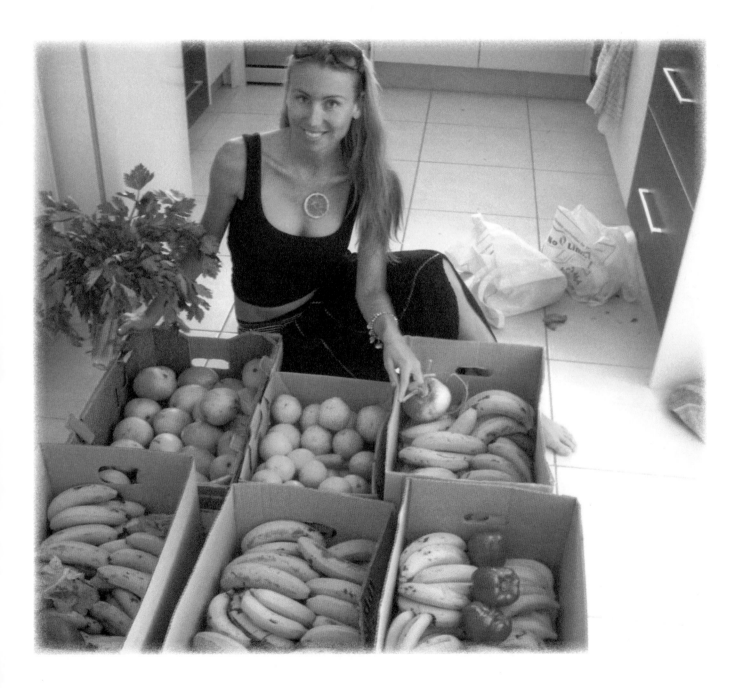

# SHOPPING LIST *week 5*

## Fruit
- ❑ 7 Bananas
- ❑ 15 Medium Peaches
- ❑ 10 Medium Figs
- ❑ 4 cups / 21 oz / 600g Grapes
- ❑ 12 dates

## Vegetables
- ❑ 1kg Organic Potatoes
- ❑ 3 Head Lettuce
- ❑ 1/2 Avocado

## Optional
- ❑ 2 Tbsp Coconut sugar

## Shelf Item
- ❑ Italian Herbs, dried
- ❑ Low Sodium Dipping Sauce
- ❑ 2 tsp Carob Powder
- ❑ Peppermint Sweet Leaf Drops
- ❑ 2 tsp Carob Powder

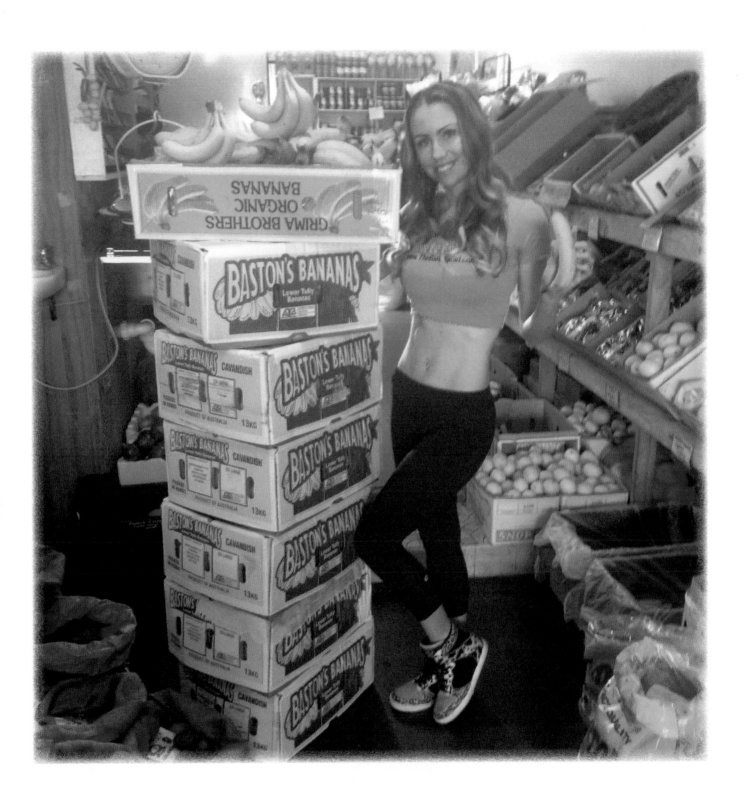

# RECIPES

Welcome to the tasty end of the book. You are about to delve into some of the yummiest, healthiest recipes on the planet! These are best RT4 approved recipes I could find. Carefully selected from my own collection and also from the wider community. These recipes not only taste delicious but are super easy to recreate. Because they are free of animal products and excess fat they will leave you feeling positive, satisfied, and guilt-free.

I've had the pleasure of including some super talented fruit lovers from instagram and youtube in this book. These peeps are responsible for a number of exceptional recipes and photos that you will find in the following pages. I love to promote those in the community who are doing amazing work and are also supportive of the Raw Till 4 lifestyle. Lettuce continue to bring this community together by promoting each others work. Please take a moment to subscribe to their pages and youtube channels, you will not regret it!

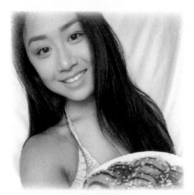

**CHERIE**

IG: thrivingonplants

youtu.be/HpdRJsjtvt4

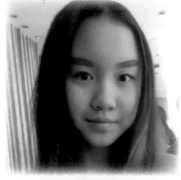

**CHELS**

IG: healthiecook

thehealthiecooklife.blogspot.com

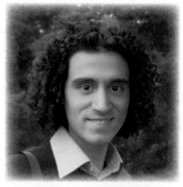

**RAOUL & MIRIAM**

IG: thevegancorner

youtube.com/user/thevegancorner

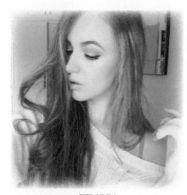

**TIANA**

IG: tianaaaxx

youtu.be/NXpZXUw-URI

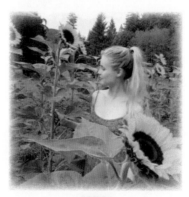

**ANNA**

IG: eat_to_thrive

youtu.be/S0WDymm9Rvl

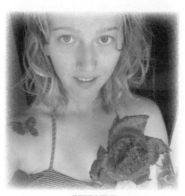

**KHADI**

IG: thevegandancergirl

youtu.be/OynLGDqL5lo

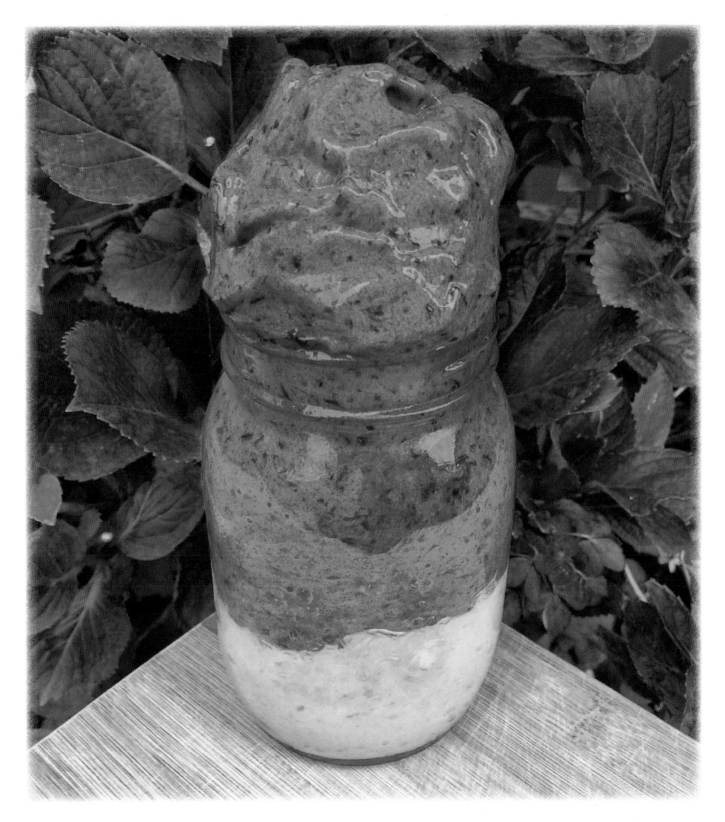

Layered Berry Nicecream - pg. 135

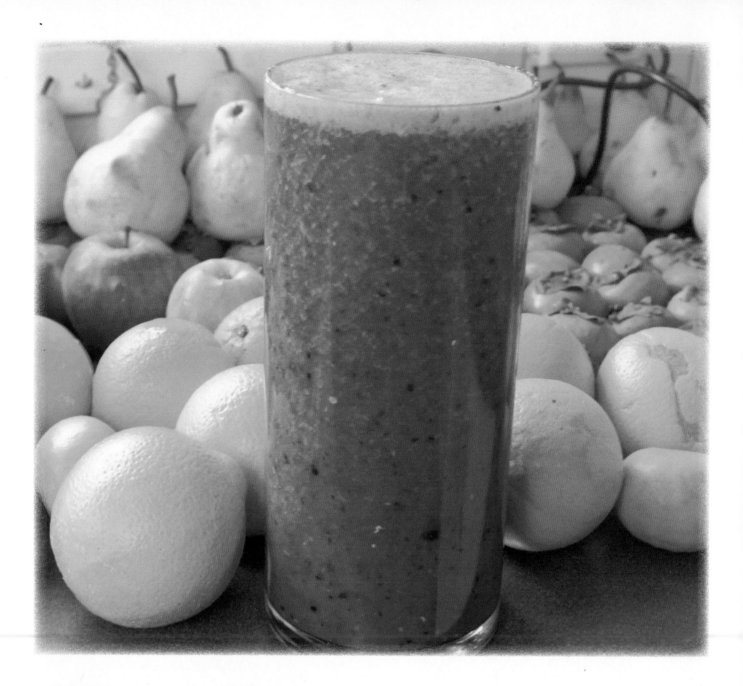

# SMOOTHIES

*For Smoothie recipes, place ingredients into the blender and blend until smooth. Banana smoothies often require pulse blending in order for them not to oxidise and become bitter. Play around with your blending technique until you get a consistency you enjoy.*

# CREAMY GREEN SMOOTHIE

*The delicious way to get your greens in! Spinach is a good source of folate, vitamin K and is a good source of insoluble fibre.*

**7 Medium Bananas**
**1/2 cup Baby Spinach**
**8 oz / 1 cup Soy Milk**
**13 oz / 400 ml Water**
**Optional: 1 tbsp Coconut Sugar**

Blend on high until desired consistency.

**Credit:** @thevegancorner

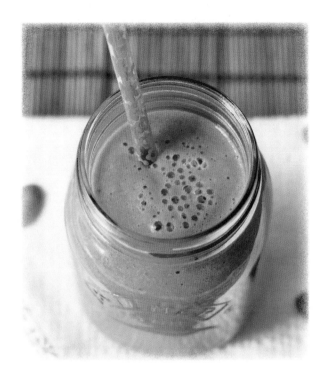

# GREEN SMOOTHIE

*Eating healthy never tasted so good, this nourishing smoothie is a winner.*

**7 Medium Bananas**
**1/2 cup Spinach**
**20 oz / 600 ml Water**
**Optional: 1 tbsp Coconut Sugar**

Blend on high until desired consistency.

**Credit:** @thevegancorner

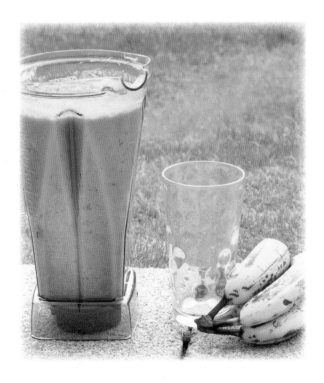

# PEPPERMINT CRISP

*Minty goodness! Carob is a tasty substitute for cocoa and the dates make it a good source of iron. It is sure to give you the energy you need!*

**10 Medjool Dates**
**1-2 Peppermint Drops or Fresh Mint**
**20 oz / 600 ml Water**
**Optional: 1 tbsp Coconut Sugar**

Blend on high for around 45 secs to 1 min, until frothy.

**Credit:** @freelee

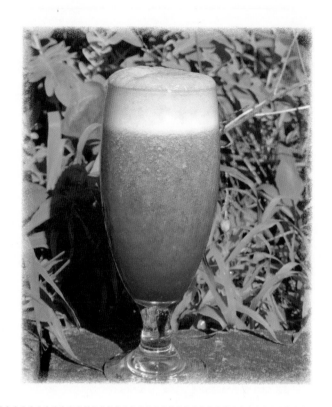

# ORANGE BERRY SMOOTHIE

*This summer time smoothie can be enjoyed all year round. Juicy oranges and berries are a match made in heaven. Oranges are known for their vitamin C, folate and calcium content so it's not just delicious but healthy!*

**10 Oranges**
**1 Cup Frozen Berries**

Juice the oranges and blend this juice with the berries. Another option is you could blend the peeled oranges and blend this with the berries, this gives a thicker/chunker version.

**Credit:** @freelee

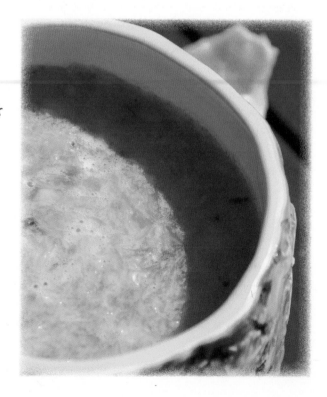

# CREAMY RT4 SMOOTHIE

*A hydrating smoothie perfect for people on the go. Coconut water is rich in B vitamins and is known for its electrolyte profile.*

**7 Medium Bananas**
**Vanilla Sweet Leaf Drops**
**8 oz / 1 cup Coconut water**
**13 oz / 400ml Water**
Optional:1 tbsp Coconut Sugar

Blend on high until desired consistency.

**Credit:** *@freelee*

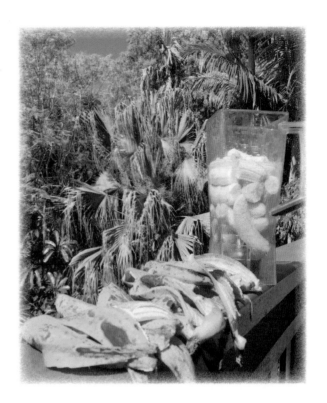

# DATEORADE

*The famous Datorade! Simplicity at its best. Dates contain iron, potassium and calcium and are a good source of insoluble fibre. They are definitely a staple in my diet.*

**12 Medjool Dates**
**20 oz / 600 ml Water**
Optional: 1 tbsp Coconut sugar

Blend on high for around 45 secs to 1 min, until frothy.

**Credit:** *@freelee*

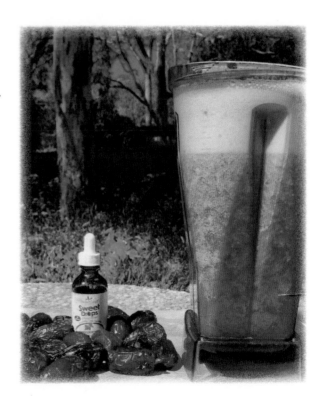

# BERRY AND COCONUT WATER REFRESHER

*This is the perfect summers drink that will keep you refreshed and energised!*

**2 cups / 16 fl oz Coconut Water**
**2 cups Mixed Frozen Berries**
**5 Medjool Dates**
**2 tbsp Coconut Sugar**
**200ml /6 fl oz Water**
**Coconut Flakes, Optional to garnish**

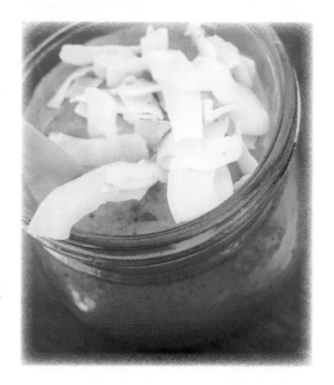

Pit the dates and place the rest of the ingredients, except for the coconut flakes, in the blender. Blend on high for around until you get your desired consistency. Serve and garnish with coconut flakes or as is.

# BANANA MANGO SMOOTHIE

*Banana and Mango is such a good combo! Mangoes contain vitamin A, folate and soluble fibre. If you can't get fresh mango just substitute with frozen.*

**5 Medium Bananas**
**1 Mango**
**8 oz / 1 cup Soy Milk**
**13 oz / 400 ml Water**
**Optional: 1 tbsp Coconut Sugar**

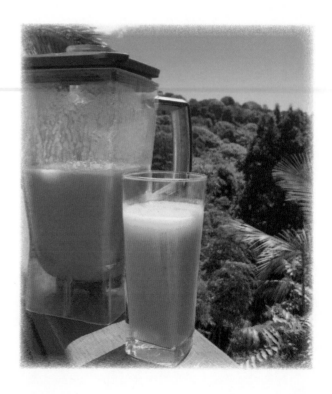

Blend on high until desired consistency.
**Credit:** *@freelee*

# APPLE PIE HUG

*Dessert in your Glass? This comforting smoothie is delicious and healthy with over 20g of insoluble fibre and an apple to keep the doctor at bay!*

**10 Medjool Dates**
**1 Apple**
**1 tsp warming spice**
**1/2 tsp cinnamon**
**20 oz / 600 ml Water**
**Optional: 1 tbsp Coconut Sugar**

Blend on high for around 45 secs to 1 min, until frothy.

**Credit:** @freelee

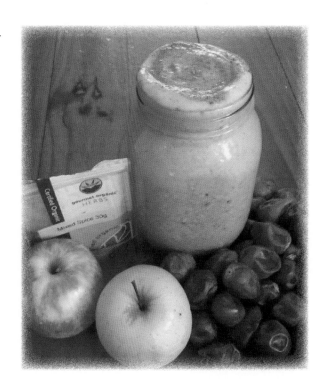

# BG BERRY BLAST

*A twist on the Datorade with berries! This is a good recipe when you haven't been shopping in a while because frozen berries and dates are easy to always have around. This is a fresh and satisfying smoothie, I hope you enjoy!*

**10 Medjool Dates**
**1 cup Mixed Frozen Berries**
**20 oz / 600 ml Water**
**Optional: 1 tbsp Coconut Sugar**

Blend on high for around 45 secs to 1 min, until frothy. Strain Seeds if desired.
**Credit:** @freelee

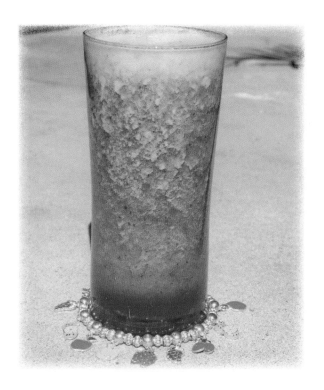

# CHOC MINT REFRESH

*Chocolate milk without the pus! A healthy version of this classic drink so enjoy it guilt free!*

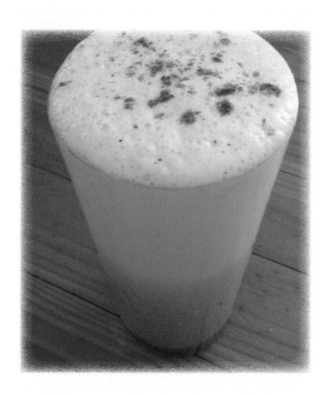

**12 dates**
**1 tbsp Carob powder**
**Peppermint Sweet Leaf Drops**
**20 oz / 600 ml Water**
Optional: 1 tbsp Coconut Sugar

Blend on high for around 45 secs to 1 min, until frothy.

**Credit:** @freelee

# BANANA DATE AND COCONUT WATER

*This is powerhouse smoothie is full of all the good stuff! Bananas, dates and coconut water are all great sources of manganese.*

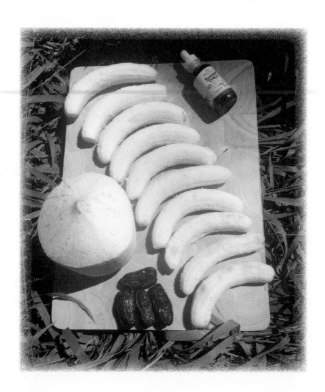

**5 Medium Bananas**
**2 Medjool Dates**
**8 oz / 1 cup Coconut water**
**13 oz / 400ml Water**
**Vanilla Sweet Leaf Drops**
Optional: 1 tbsp Coconut Sugar

Blend on high until frothy and smooth.
**Credit:** @freelee

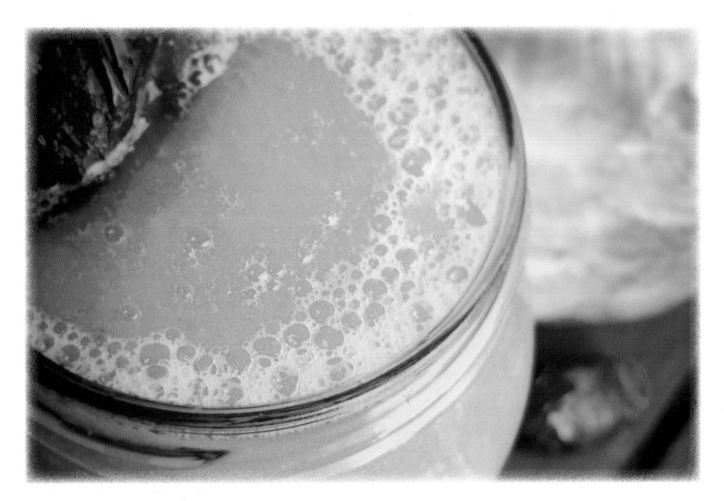

# PAPAYA DATE SMOOTHIE

*When your papayas are on point its hard to whip them into a smoothie but for every other time this is a yum combo. High in folate and ridiculously high in vitamin C, this healthy tropical fruit is refreshing and satisfying.*

**4 cups Papaya**
**8 Medjool Dates**
**20 oz / 600 ml Water**
**Optional: 1 tbsp Coconut Sugar**

Peel and deseed the papaya and place it in the blender. Remove the pits from the dates, add them to the blender along with the water and blend until smooth. For even smoother results, blend the dates first with half the water on high until smooth, then add the papaya and the rest of the water and blend.

**Credit:** *@freelee*

# KIWI PEAR AND BANANA BOMB SMOOTHIE

*The kiwi gives this smoothie a real kick, they're a good source of vitamin k and their edible seeds contain omega 3 fatty acids.*

**4 Medium Bananas**
**2 Pears**
**2 Kiwi Fruits**
**20 oz / 600 ml Water**
**Optional: 1 tbsp Coconut Sugar**

Peel the kiwi fruits and bananas. If you peel the pears the smoothie will have a smoother consistency, this is up to you, de-core the pears and place the fruit into a blender along with the other fruit and water. Pulse blend and serve.

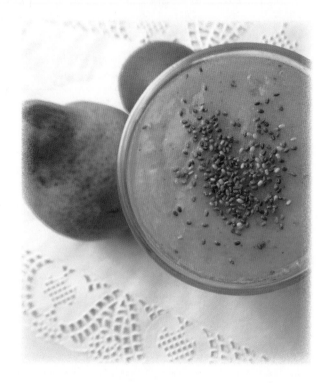

..................................................

# CREAMY BERRY DATEORADE

*A creamy berry version of Datorade.*

**10 Medjool Dates**
**1 cup Strawberries**
**8 oz / 1 cup Soy Milk**
**13 oz / 400 ml Water**
**Optional: 1 tbsp Coconut Sugar**

Blend on high for around 45 secs to 1 min, until frothy.
**Credit:** @freelee

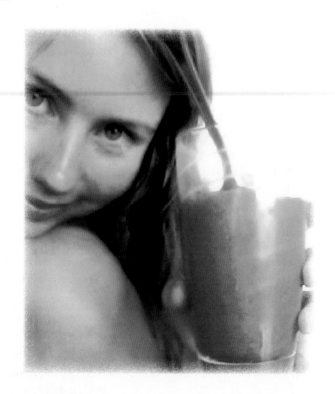

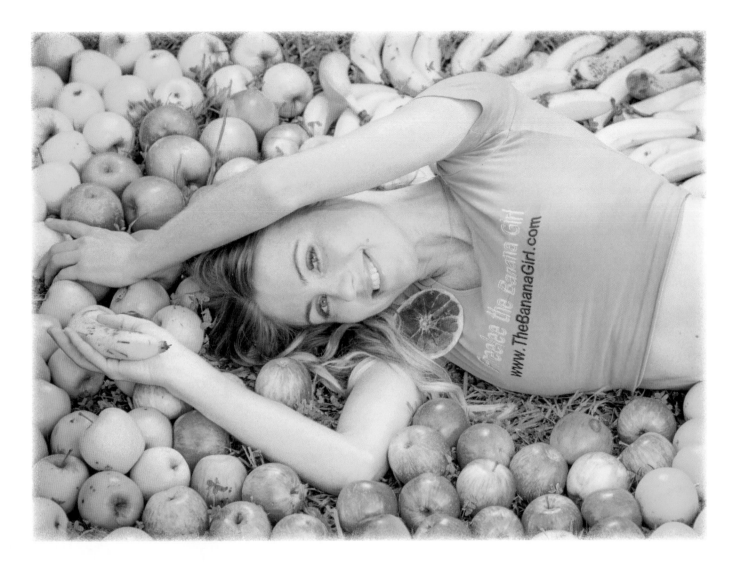

# #BGSNACKERS

*Lately I have been having this quite often, it's the perfect healthy substitute for a fatty snickers bar!*

**1-2 bananas (or just dates if no bananas)**
**10-15 Medjool Dates**
**1/2 cup to 1 cup of Vanilla Soy milk**
**1 TBSP of PB2 choc/plain peanut powder**
**1.5 litres / 50 oz water**
1 squirt of vanilla stevia drops (optional)

Blend all ingredients together till creamy and frothy.
**Credit:** @freelee

# BANANA GIRL GREEN SMOOTHIE

*The ultimate green smoothie, packed with nutrients like folate, vitamin C and iron, it is sure to make you feel good!*

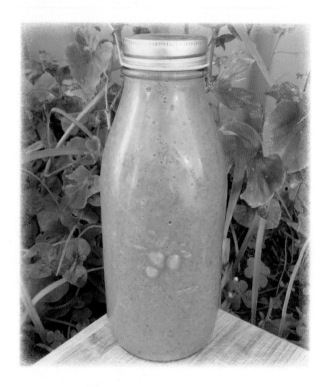

**10 Medjool Dates**
**1 cup Frozen Strawberries**
**1 cup of Baby Spinach**
**20 oz / 600 ml Water**
**Optional:1 tbsp Coconut Sugar**

Blend on high for around 45 secs to 1 min, until frothy.

**Credit:** @thrivingonplants

......................................................................

# ROCKMELON SMOOTHIE

*Rockmelon is packed with beta-carotene which is why it gives rockmelon it's orange colour. Sometimes it's just more convenient to make a smoothie than eat the fruit whole, but feel free to eat it how it comes if you like.*

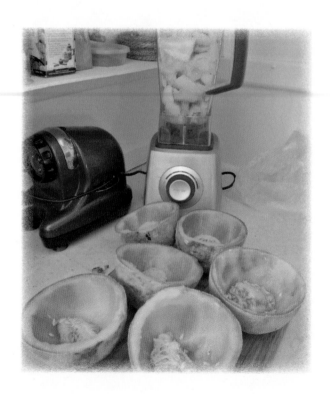

**4 Rockmelons**

Remove the edible flesh of the melon, without the seeds and add to a blender and blend on high until desired consistency.

**Credit:** @freelee

# WATERMELON JUICE

*This fruit is known for its anti-inflammatory properties as it contains a nutrient called lycopene. Watermelon juice is so refreshing but you'll need to drink a large amount if you want to get enough calories.*

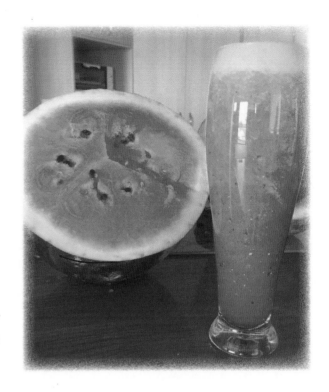

**2.4 L / 80 fl oz of watermelon juice will suffice.**

Remove the rind and put it through a juicer or blend it in a blender and sieve the the juice, if you choose to keep the fibre while blending that is fine. Also if you want to eat the fruit whole then use the following as a guide.

**15 cups / 80 oz / 2.3kg /**
**half a watermelon**
**(1 whole Watermelon which is approx 15inches x 7 inches / 38cm x 18cm)**

**Credit:** @freelee

# FRESH ORANGE JUICE

*If you've got the time and can have access to ripe oranges, enjoy a fresh glass or five.*

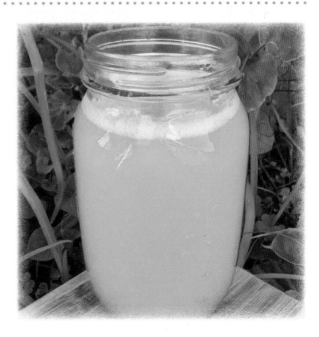

**1.5 L / 50 fl oz Fresh Orange Juice**

Juice the oranges using an electric juicer or a hand juicer.

**Credit:** @thrivingonplants

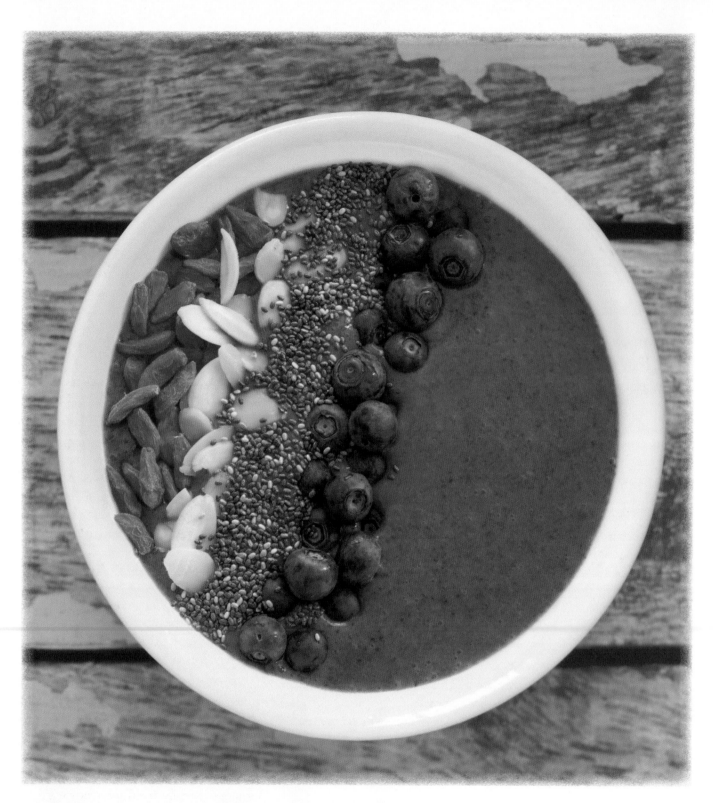

# SMOOTHIE BOWLS

# TROPICAL FRUIT SOUP

*Get excited about this tropical smoothie bowl! If you like, scape out the meat and use the coconut as a bowl.*

**4 Medium Bananas**
**1 Young Coconut - the Meat and Water**
**1 Large Papaya**
**Opt Water for Desired Consistency**

Blend the bananas, coconut meat and water, papaya with water until you reach your desired consistency, then place in either bowl coconut and enjoy the taste of the tropics.

**Credit:** @thevegandancergirl

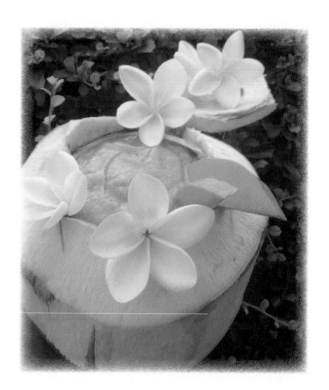

# SUMMER SMOOTHIE BOWL

*This smoothie bowl is bursting with flavour, which is no surprise when you look at the ingredients.*

**1 Large Mango**
**1/2 Large Papaya**
**4 Medium Bananas**
**2 Passion Fruits**
**Opt: 1 tbsp Coconut Sugar**

Blend the mango and papaya then ad the bananas and pulse blend the mixture. Place in a bowl and mix in the passionfruit.
**Credit:** @thevegandancergirl

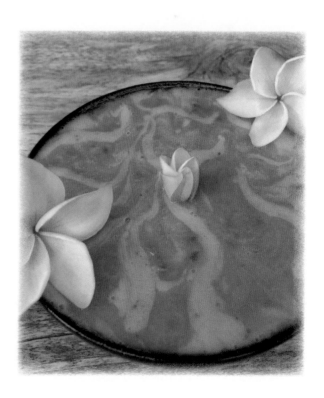

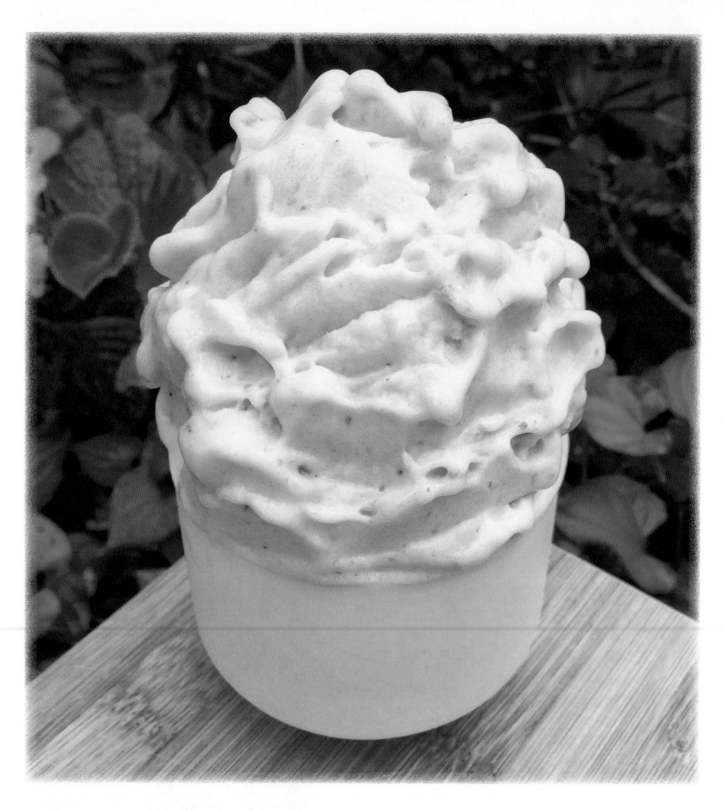

# NICE CREAMS

# BASIC BANANA NICE CREAM

Because bananas are a staple, nicecreams are a great way to eat bananas in a different way. Banana Nicecream can take on many different flavours, just add your desired flavour and enjoy! Some suggestions are vanilla, fresh mint, essence flavours and other fruits like papaya, apple etc

This is a dairy free and healthy version of everybody's favourite treat except you can eat it whenever you want guilt free!

Peel bananas and place them into a ziplock bag or tupperware container and place into the freezer for a minimum of 8 hours/overnight. (Ensure your bananas are ripe, that is, they're nice and spotty as it will allow for a much sweeter product).

Take out your frozen bananas, cut them up into approximately 2cm 'coins', put them into a food processor and pulse a few times to break up the banana chunks. Once it has broken down into a crumbly texture, turn the setting to medium/high and allow it to process until there are bits that become stuck on the sides of your processor. Open up your food processor and scrape down the edges, then continue to process. Repeat if necessary until the mixture turns smooth.

*Note: You may add a few tablespoons of water to speed up the process but if you want to keep the texture thick and creamy don't add any and just stay patient! It doesn't work as well in a blender (unless you own a high speed blender like a vitamix) as it would require more liquid whereas the food processor will slowly break down the banana into smaller pieces until it finally becomes smooth. But if all you have is a blender, not to worry, blend with whatever you have and enjoy

## 7 Frozen Medium Bananas
**Optional: 1 tbsp Coconut Sugar**

**Credit:** @thrivingonplants

# MIXED BERRY NICE CREAM

*This looks amazing, tastes amazing and the berries make it high in vitamin C, so eat up and enjoy!*

**6 Frozen Medium Bananas**
**3 Medjool Dates**
**1 cup Mixed Berries**

This recipe is the same as making Banana Nice Cream however add just the dates and berries in the blending process and Viola!

**Credit:** @thrivingonplants

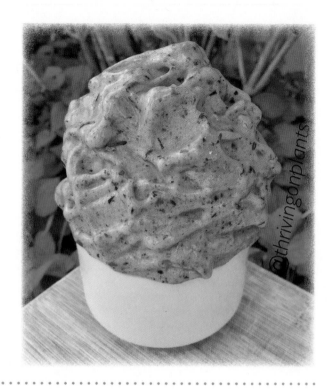

---

# BANANA NICE CREAM WITH CAROB SAUCE

*This delicious meal can be devoured guilt free. It is satisfying and begging to be eaten!*

**6 Frozen Medium Bananas**
**3 Medjool Dates**
**1 Tbsp Carob Powder**

Use the recipe for Basic Banana Nicecream

**For the Carob Sauce:**
Soak 3 dates in water overnight, or alternatively in hot water for about 5 minutes prior to use. Strain dates and add into a blender along with 2 tsp of carob powder. Blend until smooth and add in a small amount of water as needed to adjust consistency.          **Credit:** @thrivingonplants

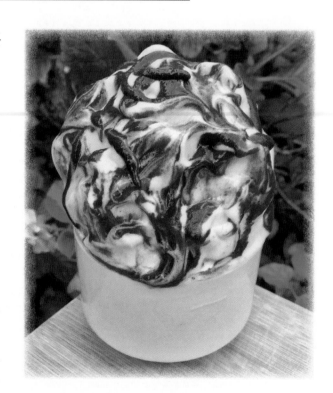

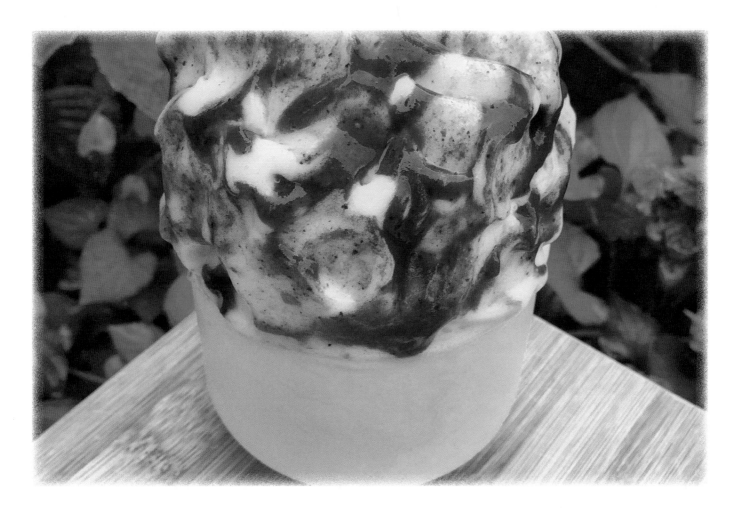

# BANANA NICE CREAM WITH BLUEBERRY SAUCE

*Bananas are also incredibly good for you, being high in healthy fruit carbohydrates they will give you the energy you need to attack your day!*

**6 Frozen Medium Bananas**
**3 Medjool Dates**
**1/2 cup frozen blueberries**

Use the recipe for Basic Banana Nicecream

**For the Blueberry Sauce:**

1. Soak 3 dates in water overnight, or alternatively in hot water for about 5 minutes prior to use. Strain dates if soaked in hot water. Add dates into a blender along with half a cup of frozen blueberries.
2. Blend until smooth, add in small amounts of water to adjust to desired consistency. Spread the sauce over a banana nice cream and enjoy.

**Credit:** @thrivingonplants

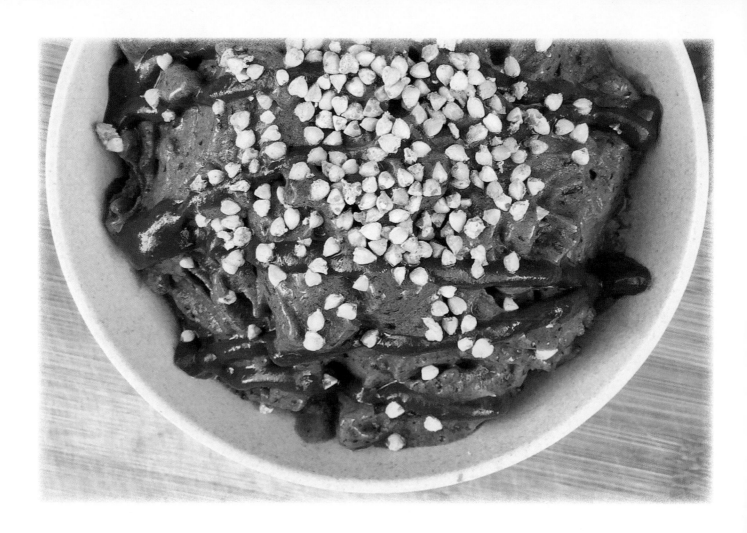

# BLUEBERRY AND BANANA NICE CREAM WITH CAROB SAUCE

*A real treat you can eat everyday! The colour and taste of this is incredible especially with that sauce.*

**6 Frozen Medium Bananas**
**1 cup Blueberries**
**3 Medjool Dates**
**2 tsp Carob Powder**
**Optional: 1 tbsp Coconut Sugar and Bukinis to garnish**

Blend your frozen bananas with the berries to make the nice cream, then use the recipe for Carob Sauce and enjoy.

**Credit:** @thrivingonplants

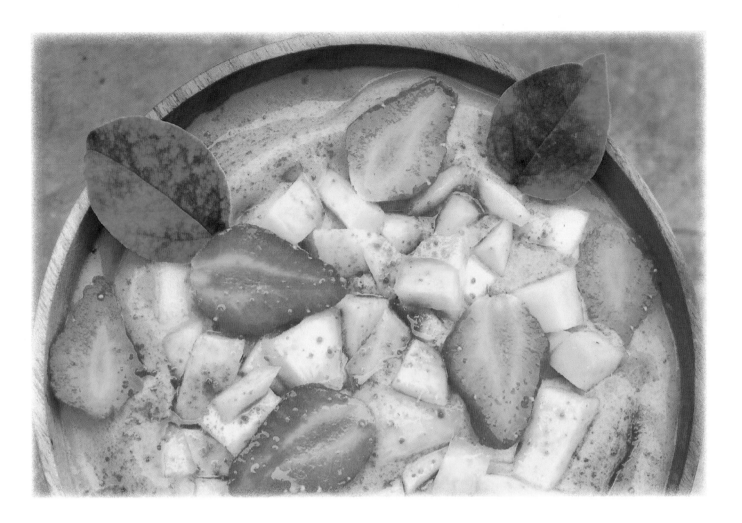

# MANGO BERRY BANANA NICE CREAM

*There is no way to get tired of fruit, when there are so many yum recipes like this one.*

**7 Frozen Medium Bananas**
**1 cup Mixed Berries**
**1 Mango**
**4 Strawberries**
**Vanilla Sweet Leaf Drops**
**Optional: 1 tbsp Coconut Sugar**

1. Put the frozen bananas (cut into small chunks), berries, and coconut sugar, into a high speed blender/food processor. Blend until it turns nice & smooth, add in the vanilla and blend again. (I don't add any water, but you can add a little if needed to help it blend).
2. Scoop into a bowl, top with the mango cubes, strawberries & extra coconut sugar! Enjoy!

**Credit:** @healthiecook

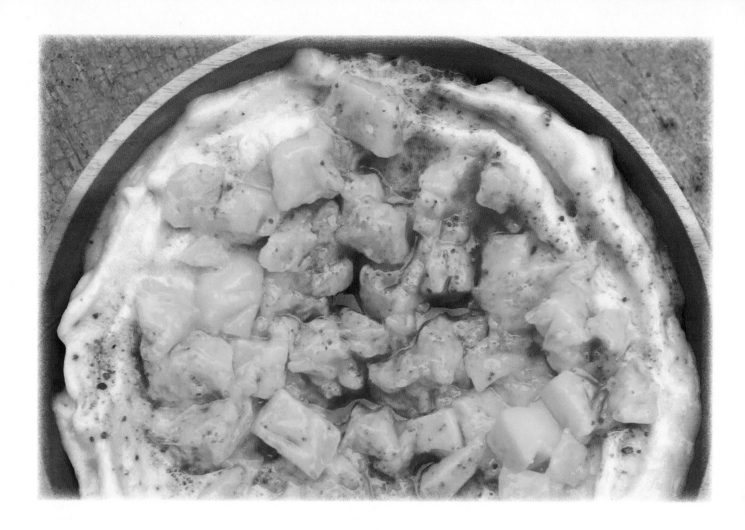

# VANILLA NICE CREAM WITH MANGO

*How delicious does this look? Adding vanilla to nice cream is a winner esp with fresh juicy mango.*

**6 Frozen Medium Bananas**
**Vanilla Sweet Leaf Drops**
**1 Mango**
**Optional: 1 tbsp Coconut sugar**

Blend the frozen bananas (cut into chunks to make it easier to blend) with the vanilla drops and optional coconut sugar. Blend on high until the mixture is smooth, add a little water gradually if needed. Scoop into a bowl and place chopped mango on top with optional coconut sugar.

**Credit:** @healthiecook

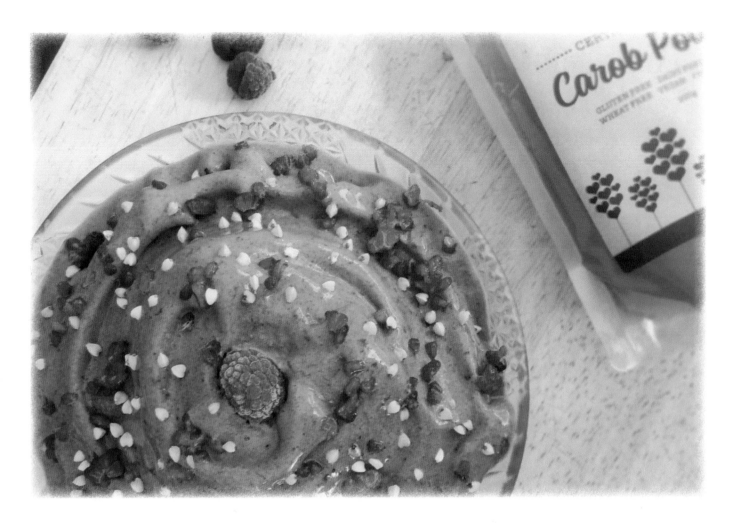

# CAROB NICE CREAM WITH RASBERRIES

*Carob and raspberries taste so well together plus carob and raspberries are both good sources of calcium.*

**7 Frozen Medium Bananas**
**1 tbls Carob Powder**
**1/2 cup of Fresh Raspberries**
**Optional: 1 tbsp Coconut sugar and bukinis**

To make the carob nice cream, just make the Basic Banana Nice Cream and add carob powder before blending. Either chop or keep your rasberries whole, add to the mix and serve.

**Credit:** @tianaaaxx

# MIXED BERRIES AND CHIA NICE CREAM

*Another day another nicecream… If you get the chance the pomegranates make it really special*

**6 Frozen Medium Bananas**
**1 cup Mixed Frozen Berries**
**4 tbsp Chia Seeds**
**Opt: 1 tbsp Coconut Sugar, Strawberries and Pomegranates**

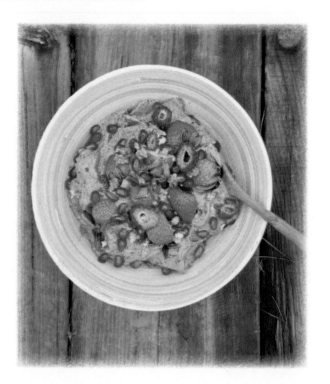

Soak the chia seeds for between 10mins to 2 hours. Make Basic Banana Nice Cream while adding the berries before blending. Add the chia seeds onto of the nicecream and as an option add strawberries and pomegranates.

**Credit:** @eat_to_thrive

# PAPAYA NICE CREAM WITH PASSIONFRUIT

*A great combination of fruits to make a great nicecream.*

**6 Medium Frozen Bananas**
**15 oz / 3 cups / 1/2 Large Papaya**
**4 Passion Fruits**
**Optional: 1 tbsp Coconut Sugar**

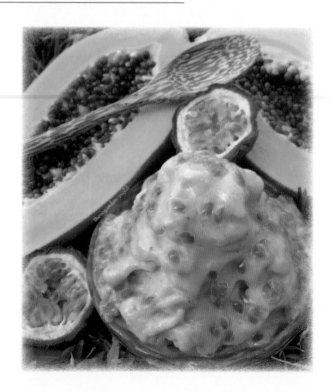

Use frozen bananas and blend them with the papaya until it is smooth. Add the passionfruit on top and serve.
**Credit:** @thevegandancergirl

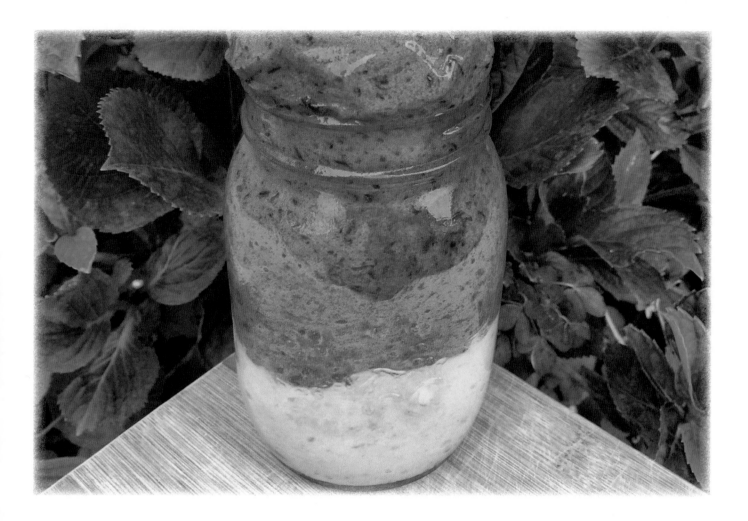

# LAYERED BERRY NICE CREAM

*This combination of berries and banana never seems to disappoint. High in health promoting antioxidants this smoothie is sure to make you look and feel good!*

**6 Frozen Medium Bananas**
**1/2 cup Mixed Frozen Berries**
**1/2 cup Frozen Strawberries**
**Optional: 1 tbsp Coconut Sugar, Vanilla Sweet Leaf Drops**

To make the first layer blend two bananas together, it is optional to add Vanilla Sweet Leaf Drops to this. Now blend another two bananas with the mixed frozen berries and then another two bananas with the frozen strawberries. Add coconut sugar to each layer if you like. Layer your dish with the three different nice creams and enjoy.

**Credit:** @thrivingonplants

# MANGO PASSIONFRUIT BANANA PARFAIT

*Sometimes you just need a layered, nicecream fruit mess in a jar. This will make you look forward to mango season but other fruits can obvs be substituted for sure.*

**4 Frozen Medium Bananas**
**2 Mangoes**
**3 Passion Fruits**
**Optional: 1 tbsp Coconut Sugar**

For the Banana Mango Nice Cream blend 1 frozen bananas with 1 large mango, you can substitute frozen mango here if you like. For the Banana Nicecream, blend 3 frozen bananas together. Peel and chop up 1 mango. Layer your dish with the two nicecreams, chopped mango and passionfruit. Add optional Coconut sugar to any layer of the parfait.

**Credit:** @thrivingonplants

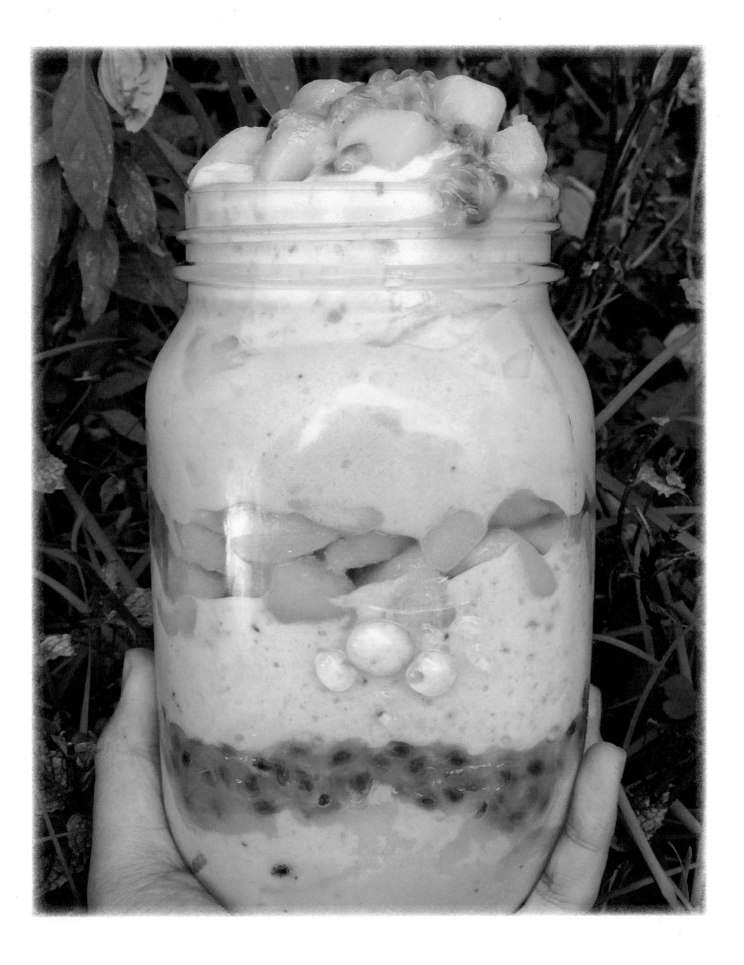

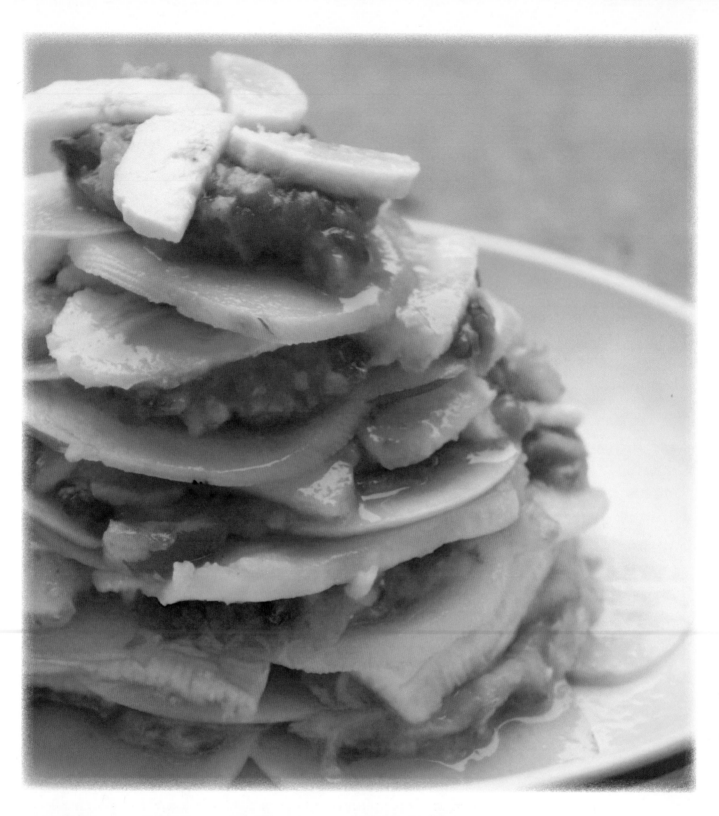

# SPECIAL RAW DISHES

# BANANA GIRL APPLE STRUDEL

*This is definitely worth the effort, when you're feeling like a raw dish that will satisfy this it is. Make it to share with a friend or better yet all for yourself.*

**1 Apple**
**3 Medium Bananas**
**6 Medjool Dates**
**Optional: Coconut Sugar / Cinnamon**

1. Take the dates, half a banana and a little grated apple, BLEND until thick and pasty (not runny). Don't add water unless you absolutely have to then only add a tiny to get the blender moving. Put paste aside.
2. Cut a banana in half then cut in thin slices lengthways (for layers). Cut/mandoline apple slices very thinly for layers.
3. Layer down slices of banana then a layer of apples followed by a layer of BAD paste (banana, apple, date). Repeat to desired height then eat before loved ones dive on it. Optional add cinnamon and/or Coconut Sugar to paste or sprinkle over.

**Credit:** @freelee

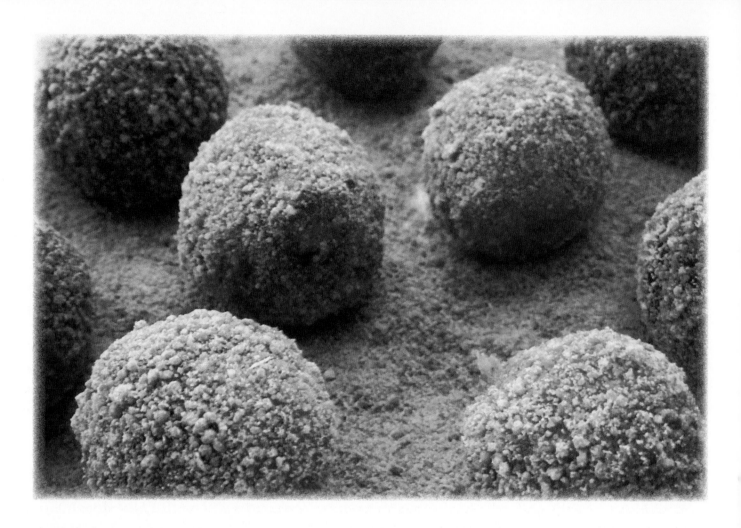

# BG BALLS

*A fun way to eat your dates, plus a great idea to keep them in the fridge for a quick go to snack.*

**12 Medjool Dates**
**Peppermint Sweet Leaf Drops**
**Optional: Coconut Sugar**

Pit the dates and place them into a food processor along with the peppermint, if you don't have one then use a blender. Spoon out the mixture one at a time and use your hands to roll into balls. Optional, roll the balls in a plate of coconut sugar to coat the surface.

**Credit:** @freelee

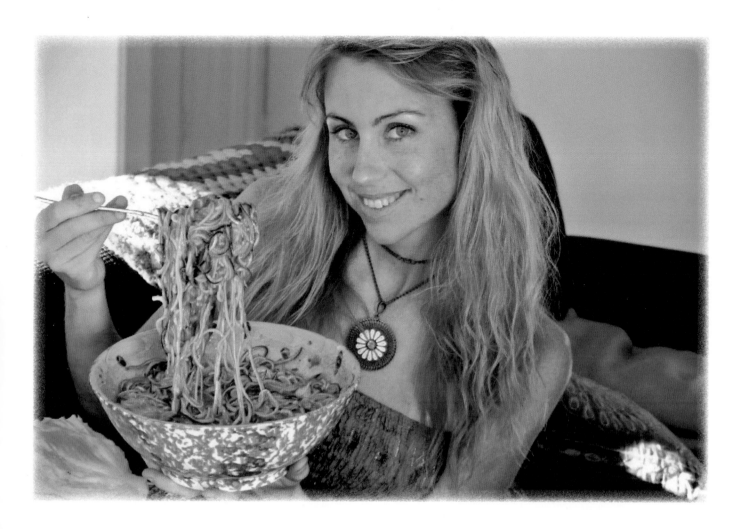

# THAI MANGO NOODLES

*A fresh raw meal bursting with flavour, this will leave you feeling raw yet satisfied. A thai version of this well known raw dish.*

**4 Large Mangoes**
**3 Zucchinis or Cucumbers**
**1/2 bunch Coriander**
**3 sprigs Thai Basil**
**1 Kafir Lime Leaf**
**0.5 cm Lemongrass**
**Optional: Chilli or chilli flakes, adjust herbs to taste**

Spiralise the zucchinis and pat dry with paper towel. Peel the mangoes, remove the seed and place the flesh with the coriander, basil, lime leaf, lemongrass and optional chilli in a blender or food processor and blend until smooth. Mix the sauce through the noodles and serve.
**Credit:** @freelee

# BG BANANA CAKE

*The ultimate fruit cake, imagine bringing this to a friends party or sharing with your family.*

**24 Medium Bananas**
**22 Medjool Dates**
**10-15 dried Turkish figs**
**1 cup of young coconut meat**
**1 cup of coconut water**
**3 drops of vanilla creme stevia drops**
**2 heaped tsps of warming spice, cinnamon, cardamom, ginger, nutmeg, cloves**

**Base:**
Process 18 dates, all figs and warming spice in food processor or blender till combined, put aside.

Grease tin with a small amount of coconut oil then dust with carob powder to provide non-stick surface for base.

**Vanilla Creme:**
Blend remaining dates with coconut flesh with half to one cup of coconut water and 3 drops of vanilla creme stevia drops until you get a smooth creamy consistency, put aside.

Press base into spring form tin then layer 2 layers of thinly sliced bananas followed by a spread of vanilla creme, continue alternating until tin is filled and have fun with the decorations!
Place in freezer or fridge for 2hrs to assist in setting the torte.

**Credit:** *@freelee*

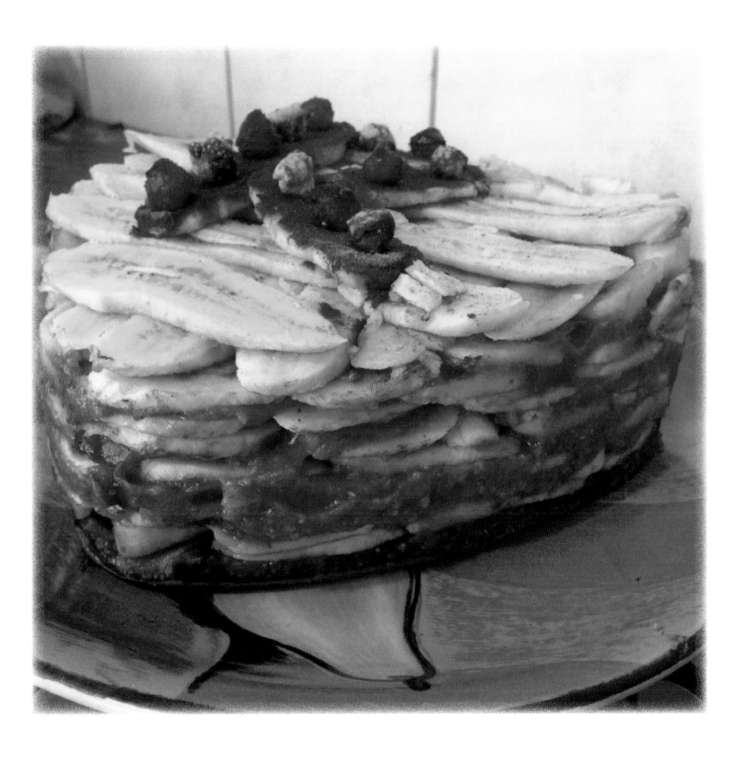

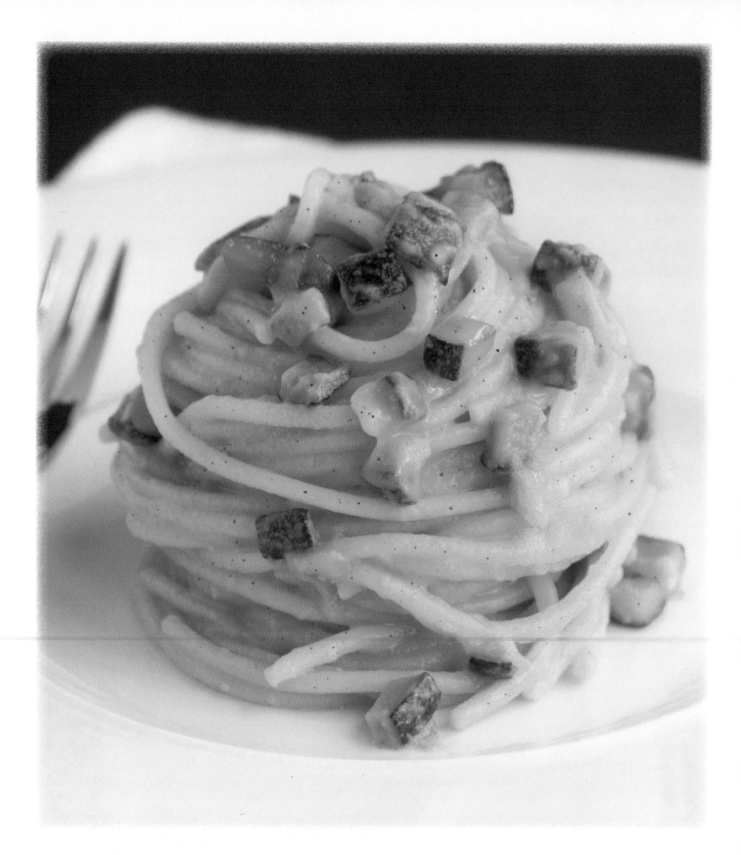

# COOKED FOOD

# PASTA ALLA CARBONARA

**7oz zucchini - 200g**
**2oz boiled carrots - 60g**
**0.5oz miso paste - 15g**
**pinch of smoked paprika**
**⅛ tsp garlic granules**
**⅛ tsp onion granules**
**1 tsp all-purpose flour - 3g**
**3 tbsp nutritional yeast - 10g/0.3oz**
**½ cup + 1 tbsp non-dairy milk - 135g/4.7oz**
**7oz uncooked spaghetti – 200g**
**Optional: salt and pepper to taste**

1. Let's start from the zucchini, which should be diced into peas-sized pieces.
2. For the sauce, place the carrots, the miso, the paprika, the garlic and onion granules, the flour, the nutritional yeast and the milk into a container, and blitz them with a stick blender to obtain a smooth and lump free sauce.
3. Now take a non-stick pan, place it over a medium heat, tip in the zucchini and cook them for roughly 10 minutes or until they become slightly golden brown. This step requires you to stir every now and then to avoid burning the vegetables, and also to allow the zucchini to brown uniformly. Once finished, turn off the heat, remove the zucchini from the pan and set them aside for later use.
4. It is now time to cook the pasta, which can be done by following to the instructions on the packet.
5. Next, place the pan back over a high heat, add in the previously prepared sauce and tip in the cooked pasta. Stir the ingredients well until the sauce thickens and coats the pasta to perfection, yielding a delicious looking final dish.
6. Now, it is time to add the zucchini back into the pan and stir them in.
7. The last two things to mention are: firstly, make sure to taste the pasta and adjust salt if desired, and secondly, carbonara cannot be called carbonara without a reasonable quantity of black pepper on it, so make sure to add it to the dish before serving it.**Credit:** @thevegancorner

# SHEPARDS PIE

## For the filling:
3oz white onion - 90g
1.5oz celery - 45g
3oz carrots - 90g
4oz mushrooms - 120g
1 garlic clove - 5g
½ tsp mixed fresh herbs - 2g
2oz peas - 60g
8oz cooked lentils - 120g
1 pinch of black pepper
1 tbsp tomato concentrate - 15g/0.5oz
1 tbsp soy sauce, low sodium - 15g/0.5oz
1 tsp cider or apple vinegar - 5g/0.2oz
¾ cup water - (180g/6.3oz)
1 tbsp all-purpose flour - 9g/0.3oz
salt to taste (if desired)

## For the topping:
14oz floury potatoes, cooked - 400g
1 pinch of black pepper
½ cup non-dairy milk - 120g/4.2oz

1. Start by chopping the onions, the celery, the carrots and the mushrooms, into peas-sized pieces, and the garlic into slices.

2. Last but not least, the herbs; simply chop them as finely as possible.

3. Next, take a no-stick pan and place it over a high heat. Tip in the celery, the carrots, the onions and the garlic, and cook them for roughly 5 minutes or until slightly softened.

4. Add the mushrooms, the peas, the lentils and the black pepper, and cook for another 2 minutes.

5. It is now time to add in the rest of the ingredients, so start by mixing in the tomato paste and then add in the chopped herbs, the soy sauce and the vinegar. Give the ingredients a good stir before moving on.

6. On the side, mix the water with the flour and add the mixture into the pan and stir. The only thing that remains to be done is to bring the liquid to a boil and reduce it down until it

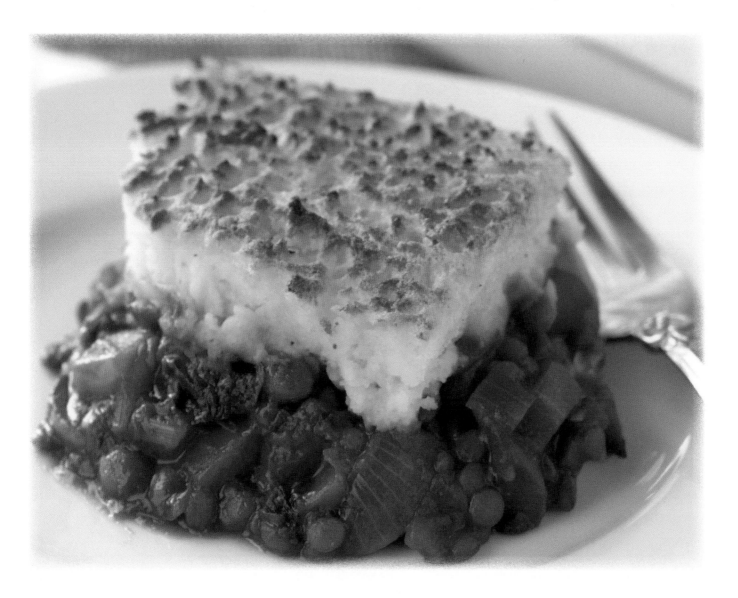

thickens and becomes of the desired consistency.

7. After that, simply let the mixture cool down completely before moving on and also remember to taste the filling and adjust the salt if desired.

8. To make the topping, start by mashing the potatoes into a bowl using a potato masher, or a fork. Add in some black pepper, the non-dairy milk, and then stir well until the mixture comes together into a sort of stiff mash.

9. To make the final pies, start by pouring the desired amount of filling into an oven dish. Then, scoop the topping over the filling to cover it completely and give the surface a little texture by piercing it with a fork. The last step is to bake the pies under the grill until the potato mash becomes golden brown. If you don't have a grill, preheat the oven to 230°C (about 450°F) and bake until golden brown. With these quantities you will be able to fill a 22x13 cm (8.5x5 inches) oven dish.

**Credit:** @thevegancorner

# PIZZA (SERVES 2)

½ cup + 3 tbsp cold water - 165g/5.8oz
¾ tsp salt - 5g/0.2oz
3 tsp sugar - 12g/0.4oz
¾ tsp instant yeast - 3g/0.1oz
2⅓ cup all-purpose/plain flour - 290g/10.2oz

## Substitution and Tips:

If you want to get perfect results at any time, make sure to use a kitchen scale. Spoons and cups are quite inaccurate and they lower the consistency of your cooking.

With this quantity of ingredients you can make a pizza that is roughly 25x35cm (10x14 inches) large.

Instant yeast, also known as bread machine yeast, is the kind to be added directly to dry ingredients, but it can also be dissolved directly into the water.

Salt can be avoided if not desired. However, you should know that it has a retarding effect on the activity of the yeast, so if you don't plan on using it, expect your pizza to rise in a shorter amount of time.

If you want to use a gluten free flour you can, just expect slightly different results

1. To begin with, place the water, the salt and the sugar into a bowl large enough to accommodate all the ingredients. Whisk the ingredients to dissolve the sugar and the salt.
2. Now add in the yeast and whisk again to dissolve it into the water.
3. Add the flour into the bowl all at once and mix the ingredients together with a spatula until you obtain a rough dough.
4. Transfer the rough dough onto a working surface and knead it by hand for 2 minutes until it becomes smooth and soft to the touch. In case you find the dough to be too sticky, you can add a little more flour. However, try not to add too much flour or you will end up with a tough final pizza.
5. Form a ball with the dough, cover it with a bowl and let it rest for 20 minutes before moving on.
6. Once the time has elapsed, remove the bowl, dust some flour onto the dough and start rolling it down using a rolling pin.
7. You want to obtain a flat shape of the same size of the pan you are going to use, and the dough should be roughly half a centimetre thick, or a fifth of an inch.
8. To prevent the pizza from getting stuck to the tray during the cooking process, make sure to use a non-stick tray.

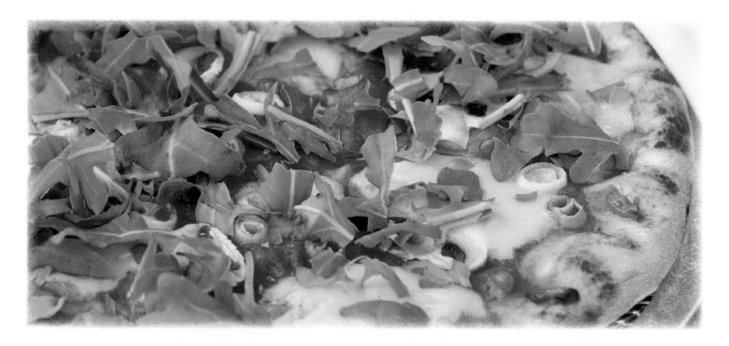

9. Now, simply move the pizza dough onto the tray, and gently press it down by hand, until it perfectly matches with the surface of the tray.

10. The next step is to pierce the entire surface of the pizza using a fork, which will allow for a more even rising. Once the pizza has been rolled down, pierced and covered, it is time for it to rise until roughly double in size, a process that will take approximately 2 hours, depending upon the temperature of the environment and the quantity of salt used.

11. To keep the surface of the pizza moist during the rising time, cover the tray with a damp kitchen towel, making sure that it doesn't come into contact with the pizza.

12. Now, place the tray in a warm place, and leave it there for the duration of the rising time.

13. 30 minutes before the time has elapsed, preheat it to 250°C or 480°F.

14. Once the time is up, and the pizza is roughly doubled in size, you can begin with the cooking process, so uncover the tray, place it into the oven and cook the pizza for exactly 3 minutes. You don't want to add any topping to the pizza during the first part of the cooking process.

15. Once the first part of the cooking time is up, remove the pizza from the oven and you'll find yourself in front of a soft and pillowy piece of bread. The first thing to do, is to spread a good layer of tomato sauce onto the base.

16. At this point, you can add any other favourite topping, including any plant-based mozzarella or cheese.

17. Once all the toppings have been added, simply place the tray back into the oven and bake the pizza for the last 4 minutes to complete the recipe. After this time, you'll have yourself an amazing homemade pizza, with a superb soft consistency and loads of flavour.

**Credit:** @thevegancorner

# PIZZA SAUCE

*This sauce can also be used as a condiment for pasta. To do this, cook it for about 10 minutes in total, tip in the cooked pasta, mix and enjoy.*

**⅛ tsp baking soda (sodium bicarbonate)**
**⅛ tsp salt (if desired)**
**1 can plum tomatoes - 400g/14oz**
**¾ tsp Italian herb mix, or oregano**

1. To begin with, place the salt and the baking soda into a container.
2. Once that's done, add in the tinned tomatoes. The baking soda is used only to lower the acidity of the tomatoes, so if you can find tomatoes that are not too acidic, you can skip this ingredient as it is not really needed.
3. Now simply blend the ingredients using a stick blender. You don't want to keep blitzing at all time, but simply process the sauce just enough to break the tomatoes apart.
4. Next, place a pan over a medium heat, add in the tomato sauce, the herbs and stir to combine the ingredients.
5. As soon as the mixture reaches the boiling point, turn the heat down to low and let the sauce simmer for 6 minutes to complete the preparation.
6. Once the cooking time has elapsed, you'll have yourself a perfect pizza sauce. You can now turn off the heat and let the sauce cool down completely before using it.

**Credit:** @thevegancorner

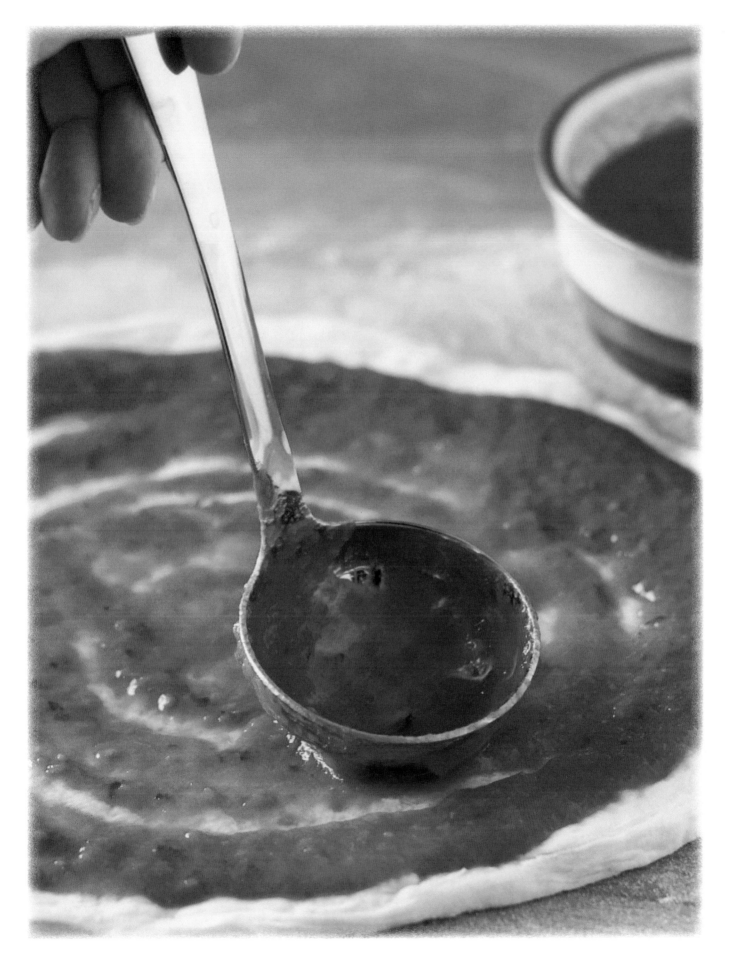

# MOZZARELLA

**1.4oz tofu - 40g**
**1 cup non-dairy milk - 240g/8.5oz**
**2 tbsp + 2 tsp tapioca starch - 20g/0.7oz**
**½ tsp salt (if desired) - 3g/0.1oz**
**1 small clove of garlic - 3g/0.1oz**

### Substitution and Tips:

Tapioca starch can be easily found in any good Asian store. The quantity and type of starch can be adjusted to obtain mozzarellas of different consistencies. For a more liquid cheese, use 18g (1 tbsp + 1 tsp) of cornstarch, and for a very elastic mozzarella, use 22g (1 tbsp + 2 tsp) of tapioca starch. To get a smoked version, add 1tsp (2g) of smoked paprika into the recipe.

You can substitute the tofu with 40g/1.4oz of one of the following ingredients: boiled potatoes, coconut cream, boiled carrots, tahini, or any favourite nuts.

This serving size of mozzarella suits the servings size of the pizza recipe in this section.

1. To begin with, place all the ingredients into the jug of a blender, and blend at high speed for roughly 30 seconds to obtain a smooth liquid.
2. Once the ingredients are properly blended, place a non-stick pan onto a medium heat and pour in the blended mixture.
3. Start stirring the sauce and keep doing so until it thickens into the final cheese. If you see some lumps forming at first, don't worry! As soon as the sauce begins to thicken properly, the lumps will dissolve into a creamy molten cheese consistency. However, to make this happen, make sure to stir vigorously as the sauce thickens.
4. You want to cook the sauce just until it begins to boil, and after that, you can turn off the heat and cool it down completely before using it.
5. Once cool, simply use the mozzarella as you please, knowing full well that it will make the most amazing plant-based pizza topping ever.

**Credit:** @thevegancorner

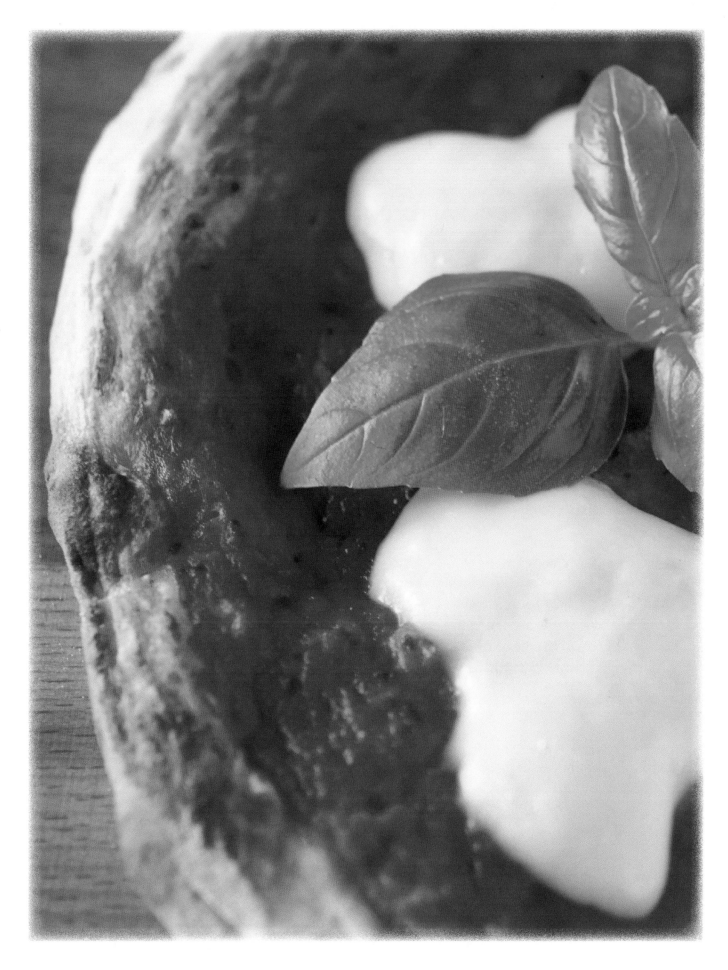

# HUMMUS

**6.5oz cooked chickpeas - 180g**
**2 tbsp + 1 tsp lemon juice - 35g/1.2**
**2.5oz silken tofu - 80g**
**1 tbsp + 2 tsp tahini - 25g/0.9oz**
**½ tsp salt - 3g/0.1oz**
**Optional: 1 small garlic clove**

## Substitution and Tips:

The tahini is a fundamental piece of the puzzle as its nutty flavour really makes a difference. For this reason, we didn't completely remove it, but simply diminished its quantity as much as possible to still obtain a great final spread. This makes this hummus not a completely fat-free version, but simply a lowfat one, which has a third of the fat of any other reduced fat hummus available on the market.

The quantity of salt mentioned in the ingredients is to obtain a hummus that tastes like the store-bought one, so you might want to add it a little at the time until you reach the right level of savouriness.

1. The recipe is pretty simple; place all the ingredients into a food processor and blitz for roughly 3 minutes or until the hummus is as smooth as you desire. If the blades don't catch all the ingredients at first, simply scrape the sides of the container with a spatula and blitz again.

**Credit:** @thevegancorner

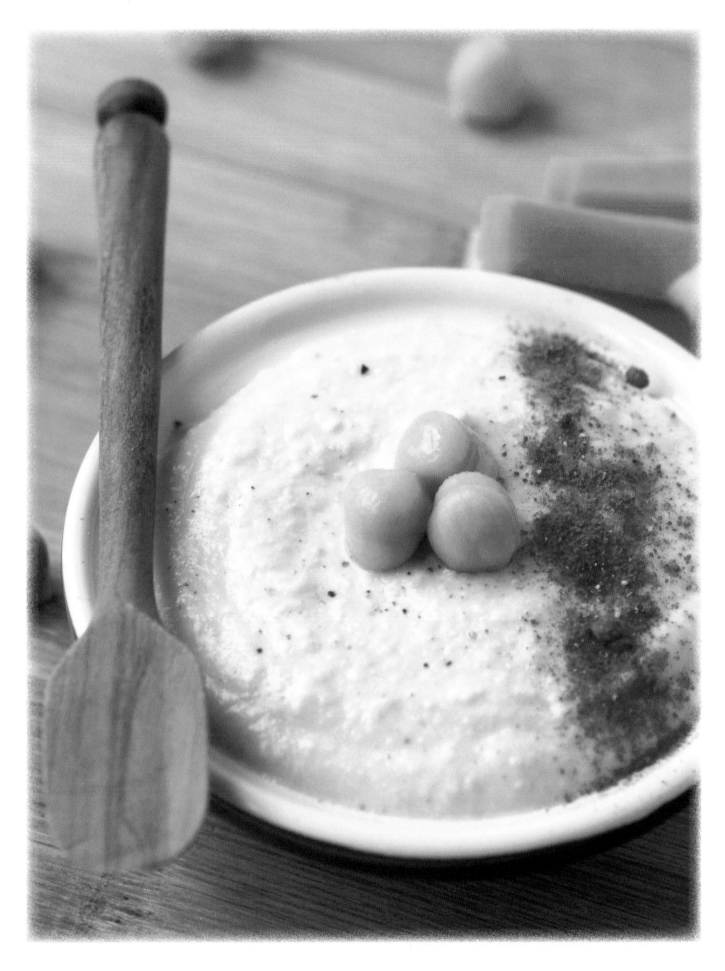

# ASIAN STYLE NOODLES

10.5oz mixed vegetables - 300g
1 tsp sugar – 4g
1 cup of vegetable stock, or water - 240g/8.5oz
2 tsp corn starch - 6g/0.2oz
1⅓ tbsp soy sauce, low sodium - 20g/0.7oz
5.3oz uncooked rice noodles - 150g
salt (if desired)

## Substitution and Tips:

You can use any noodle you prefer for this dish and you can also use any of your favourite vegetables. A good combination is mini corn, snap-peas, red bell pepper, onions and broccoli.

1. To begin with, let's prepare the vegetables. Simply cut them into strips or dice them.
2. Now, place a non-stick pan over a medium heat, add in the vegetables, the sugar and 3 tbsp of the stock (45g/1.6oz). Cook the veggies for roughly 5 minutes or until they have the the desired crunch.
3. Next, mix the rest of the stock with the starch and add it into the pan with the vegetables, followed by the soy sauce.
4. Stir well to combine and bring the ingredients to the boil. As soon as the liquid reaches boiling point, you can turn off the heat and prepare the noodles as instructed on the packet.
5. Now, return the pan onto a high heat, drain the cooked noodles and add them into the pan.
6. Start stirring to properly combine the ingredients together and obtain the ultimate delicious-looking and luscious noodles dish. This is also the right moment to taste the noodles and add salt if desired.

**Credit:** @thevegancorner

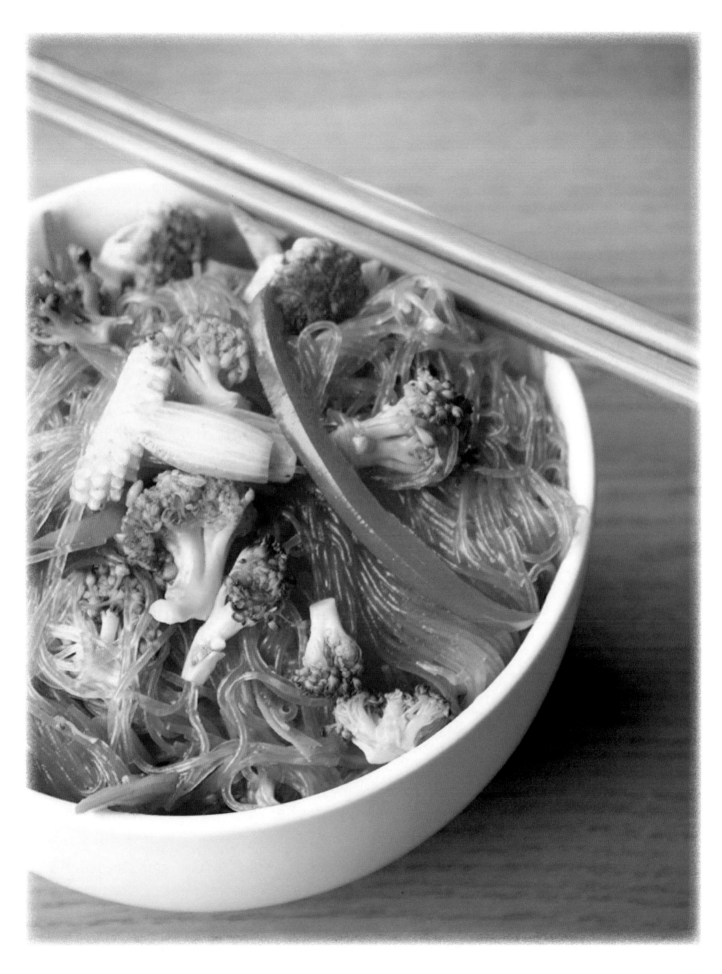

# PASTA NAPOLETANA

*There are two version of the pasta sauce, one is a homemade style and the other is a quicker and more convenient version as it's just from a jar.*

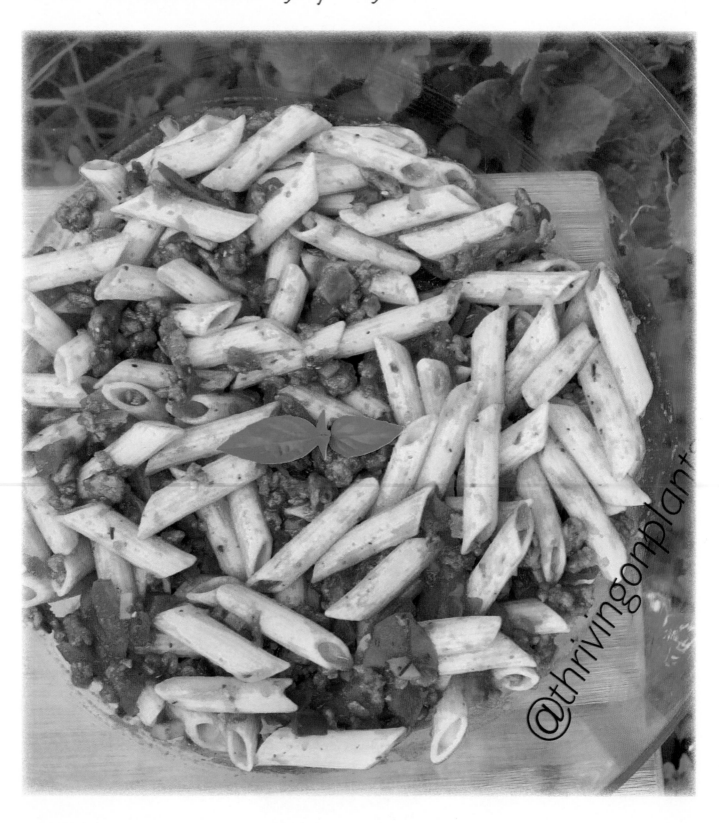

# HOMEMADE STYLE

**100 grams dry of Organic Corn Pasta - Gluten Free**
**1 can of Tomatoes**
**1 tbsp Tomato Paste (100%)**
**1/2 cup canned Lentils**
**1 cup Mushrooms**
**1/2 Head Lettuce**
**Optional: Baby spinach and your favourite spices; garlic powder, dried basil, mixed herbs and chilli flakes.**

1. Cook your pasta according to the packet instructions.
2. In a saucepan on medium, heat up a few tbsp of water, add in chopped mushrooms and saute for a few minutes until wilted. Add in your desired herbs and spices and a tbsp of tomato paste and a can of canned tomatoes. Once the water comes to the boil, lower to low/med, add the lentils and simmer until the sauce thickens.
3. Turn off the heat and add in a handful of baby spinach (the residual heat will wilt the spinach nicely). Drain pasta once cooked, top with the pasta sauce and serve with lettuce.

. . . . . . . . . . . . . . . . . . . . . . . . . . . . . . . . . . . . . . . . . . . . . . . . . . . . . . . . . . . . . . . . . . . . . . . . . . . . .

# EASIER STYLE

**100 grams dry of Organic Corn Pasta - Gluten Free**
**1/2 cup Tomato Based Pasta Sauce - Low Fat, Low Sodium**
**1/2 cup canned Lentils**
**1 cup Mushrooms**
**1/2 Head Lettuce**
**Optional: Baby spinach and your favourite spices; garlic powder, dried basil, mixed herbs and chilli flakes.**

1. Cook your pasta according to the packet instructions.
2. In a saucepan on medium, heat up a few tbsp of water, add in peeled and chopped mushrooms and drained lentils, saute for 5 minutes, occasionally stir to prevent burning. Add in the pasta sauce with your desired herbs and spices and cook for another 2 minutes or until the pasta sauce is warm.
3. Drain pasta once cooked, top with the pasta sauce and serve with lettuce.

**Credit:** @thrivingonplants

# SUSHI

*The most famous Japanese food outside of Japan. Sushi is fun to make and allows you to create whatever flavours suit you best. Choose your favourite veggies and make a meal which is fun to share or easy to take out when you're on the run.*

**3/4 cup Dry Rice**
**Nori Rolls**
**1 small Carrot**
**1 small Cucumber**
**1 small Red Pepper**
**1/2 cup Avocado**

1. Cook rice according to packet instructions. Allow rice to cool at room temperature.
2. Place 1 nori sheet (you'll need at least 4 for this recipe) shiny side down onto a sushi mat. The nori sheets have horizontal line, that will help you roll it up. Wrapping your sushi mat in some cling wrap will allow for an easier job of rolling and minimal mess. If you don't have a sushi mat, don't worry, just roll the sushi with your hands the best you can. Spread the rice evenly over the nori in a thin layer, leaving about 2cm/1inch uncovered at the far end of the nori roll.
3. Place strips of your desired filling in the centre of your rice. Beginning with the edge closest to you, use the sushi mat to roll it up firmly with even pressure. Open the mat, dab the 2cm/1inch uncovered part of the nori sheet with water and roll once again to seal the edge.
4. Cut to serve if desired, eat as is or serve with desired dipping sauce (Keep it low-sodium)

**Credit:** @thrivingonplants

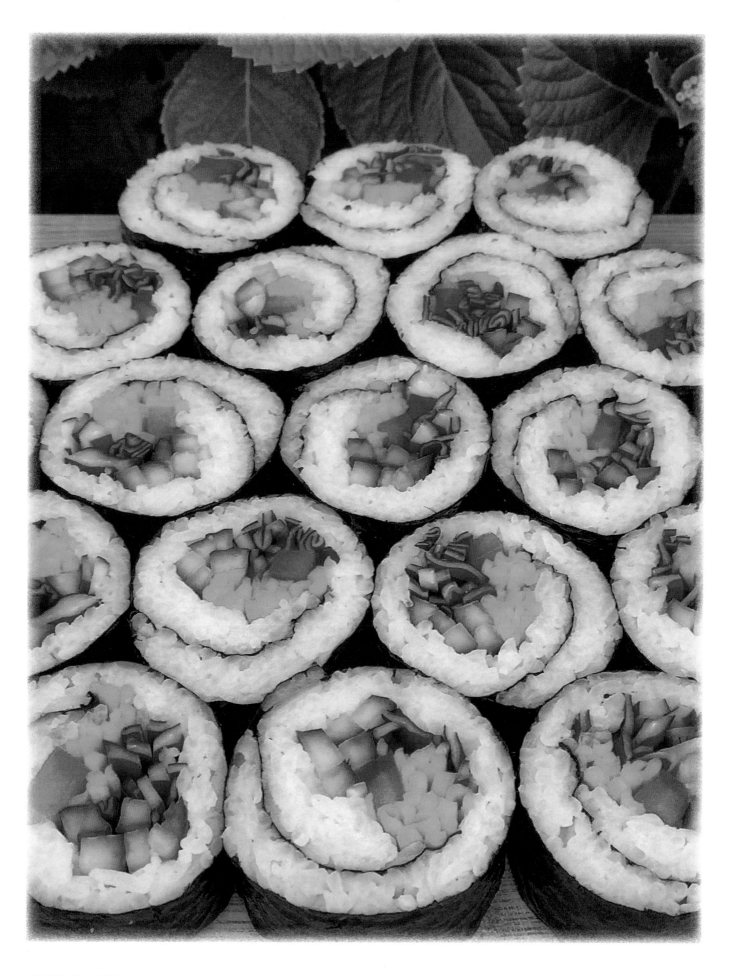

# SWEET POTATO FRIES

*A sweet variation of classic fries, these baked sweet potatoes have practically no fat. Their sweetness makes them extra satisfying plus they contain high amounts of vitamin A, try to seek out organic when possible.*

**500g Organic Sweet Potatoes**
**Sweet Chilli Sauce - Low Sodium**
**1/2 Head Lettuce Leaves**

1. Preheat oven to 220 degrees C/430 degrees F
2. Line a baking tray with non-sticking baking paper.
3. Wash potatoes thoroughly, cut into fries and pat dry. If you want to add more flavour place them into a large bowl and add desired herbs and spices. Some suggestions are 1 tsp of mixed Italian herbs, paprika, onion powder, curry powder or garlic powder etc. If preferred without the skin, peel and wash before patting dry and adding to bowl.
4. Spread the fries onto the baking tray in one single layer. Try to ensure that they aren't all touching as they won't be able to become crispy.
5. Place into preheated oven and bake for approximately 20 minutes on one side and 15 minutes on the other. The cooking time will change depending on the thickness of your fries, keep an eye on them so they don't become over crispy i.e. black.
6. Serve with lettuce and dipping sauce.

**Credit:** @thrivingonplants

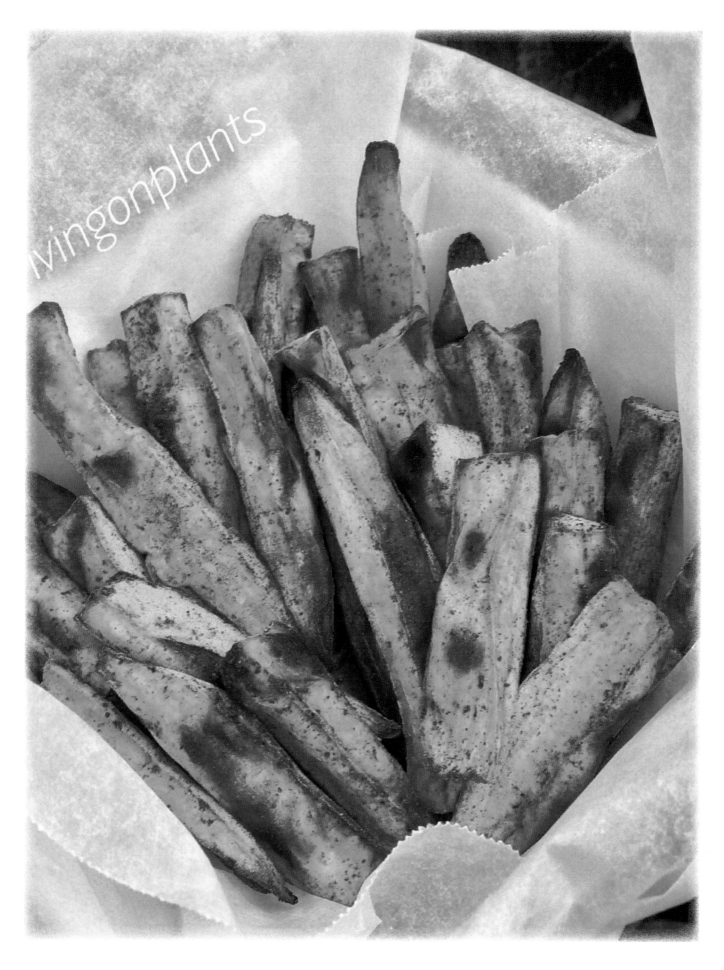

livingonplants

# #BG FRIES

*The perfect Raw Till 4 dinner. Banana Girl Fries is one of the first dishes I created when I reintroduced cooked food to my diet. Since then it has become a staple and there has been hundreds of RT4 chip recipes created for you to try. Cherie shows you how simple it is! They are incredibly satisfying, simple on digestion and you can make different versions of this staple recipe.*

**500g of Organic Potatoes**
**Low Sodium Dipping Sauce**
**1/2 Head Lettuce**

1. Preheat oven to 220 degrees C/430 degrees F
2. Line a baking tray with non-sticking baking paper.
3. Wash potatoes thoroughly, cut into fries and pat dry. If you want to dd more flavour place them into a large bowl and add desired herbs and spices. Some suggestions are 1 tsp of mixed Italian herbs, paprika, onion powder, curry powder or garlic powder etc. If preferred without the skin, peel and wash before patting dry and adding to bowl.
4. Spread the fries onto the baking tray in one single layer. Try to ensure that they aren't all touching as they won't be able to become crispy.
5. Place into preheated oven and bake for approximately 20 minutes on one side and 15 minutes on the other. The cooking time will change depending on the thickness of your fries, keep an eye on them so they don't become over crispy i.e. black.
6. Tip: If you buy a convection oven with wire tray often you do not have to turn them at all! That's exactly what I use these days.

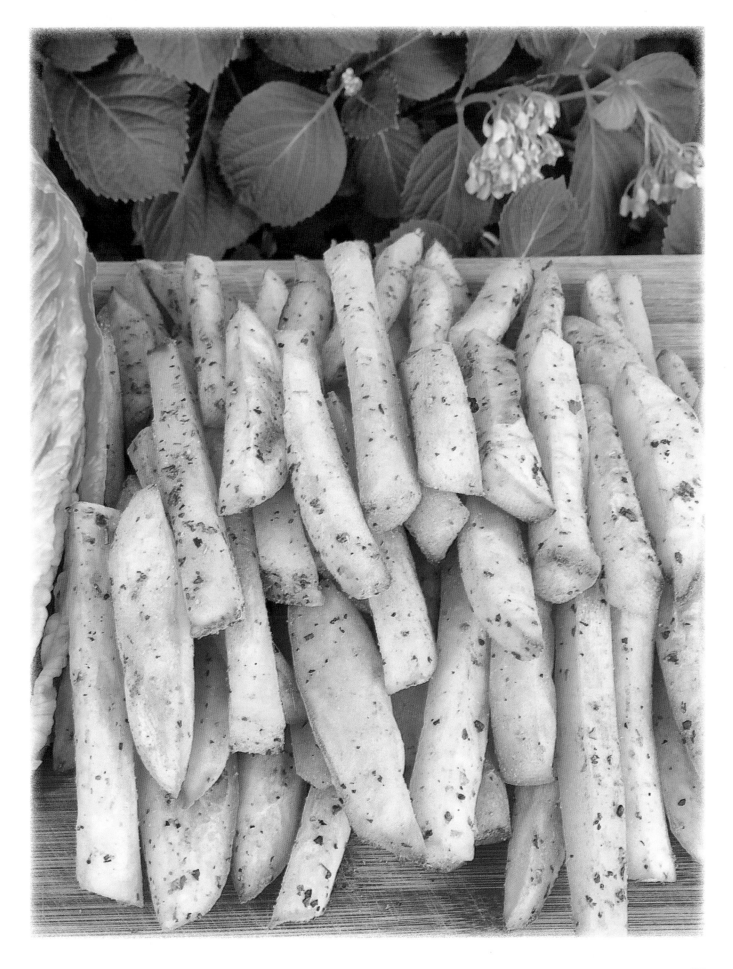

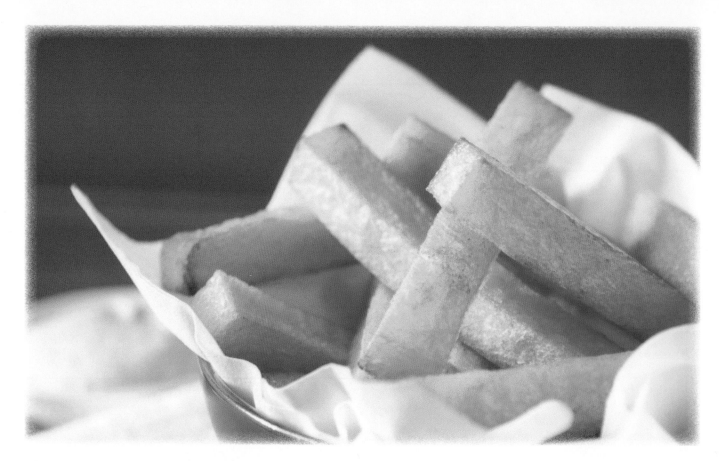

# POLENTA FRIES

**Polenta, cooked and cooled down - 600g/1.3lb per person**

1.  To begin with Preheat the oven to 220°C, which is about 430°F.
2.  To make the chips, you need a block of polenta ready to be sliced. This can be done by cooking some instant polenta, pouring it into a square container and letting it cool down completely until it solidifies.
3.  At this point, you simply want to slice the polenta and then cut the slices into chunky fries-sized pieces, roughly 1cm (or half an inch) thick.
4.  Now, all you need to do is to place those beautiful fries onto a baking tray lined with a baking mat, place the tray into the oven and bake the fries for exactly 15 minutes.
5.  Once the time has elapsed, remove the tray from the oven and you will see that the fries begin to caramelise and to crisp up a bit. To obtain a more uniform browning, flip the fries bottom side up and bake for another 15 minutes to complete the dish.
6.  Before serving you can sprinkle the fries with some salt, or eat them as they are with your favourite sauces.

**Credit:** @thevegancorner

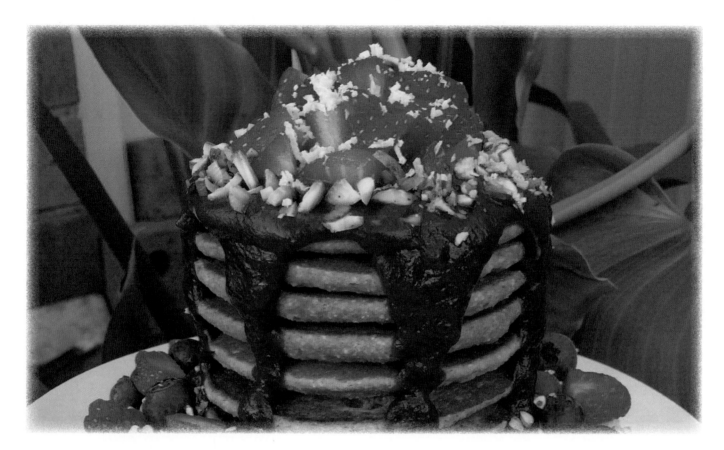

# PANCAKES

**4.2 oz / 120 g / 1.5 cup Quick Oats**
**8 oz / 1 cup Almond Milk**
**1 Banana**
**1/2 tsp Cinnamon**
**2-3 Dates**
**1-2 tbsp Carob**
**Optional: 1 tbsp Coconut Sugar and 3 tbsp Rice Malt Syrup**

## Pancake batter:

In a blender, place 1.5c quick oats ground into a flour, 1c unsweetened almond milk, 1 ripe banana, cinnamon and 1tbsp coconut sugar (I preheated my non-stick frypan on low heat before pouring in the batter and just kept it on low heat the entire time).

## Sauce:

2-3 dates, 1-2tbsp carob powder, a few tbsp water to adjust consistency OR you can simply mix rice malt syrup with the powder of your choice until it becomes a smooth sauce consistency.

**Credit:** @thrivingonplants

# SPICY ASIAN FIRE ROASTED TOFU

**1/2 of a 14-16 oz block of firm tofu**
**1 heaped tbsp Asian hot sauce (I recommend either Gochujang or Sriracha)**
**1 tbsp maple/coconut syrup**
**1 tbsp tomato paste (or use more hot sauce if you're brave/really like spicy food :p)**
**1 tsp soy sauce/tamari/less sodium**
**water, as needed**
**Optional:1/4 tsp white pepper powder**
**1/4 tsp black pepper powder**
**1/4 tsp garlic powder (or grate in 1 small clove)**
**200g of vegetables such as broccoli, bok choy, mushrooms etc**
**1 cup dry rice, cook according to package instructions, to serve**

1. First you need to prepare the tofu. Drain the liquid, wash the tofu, cut it in half lengthwise. Put a thick layer of paper towel on a plate/surface, put your tofu on there, cover with more paper towel. Put something heavy (a frying pan/wood cutting board/etc) on top and let it sit for a few minutes until the water is absorbed. After that, cut the tofu into cubes.

2. In a small bowl, whisk together all the marinade ingredients, add enough water to form a thick-pourable sauce consistency. Carefully (don't break the tofu haha) mix the tofu with the marinade in an airtight container/ziplock bag. Refrigerate overnight/at least for a few hours.

3. Preheat the oven to 180 Celcius. Line a baking sheet with parchment paper.

4. Arrange the tofu cubes (make sure none of them are touching!), spoon the leftover marinade on top of each slice. Bake for 25-30 minutes until cooked, crisp on the outside, with some caramelised parts! Don't forget to flip them halfway through.

5. Serve with a big pile of rice, some oil-free stir-fried veggies, and there you have a delicious & easy Asian style meal that's delicious, high carb low fat, and vegan of course.

**Credit:** *@healthiecook*

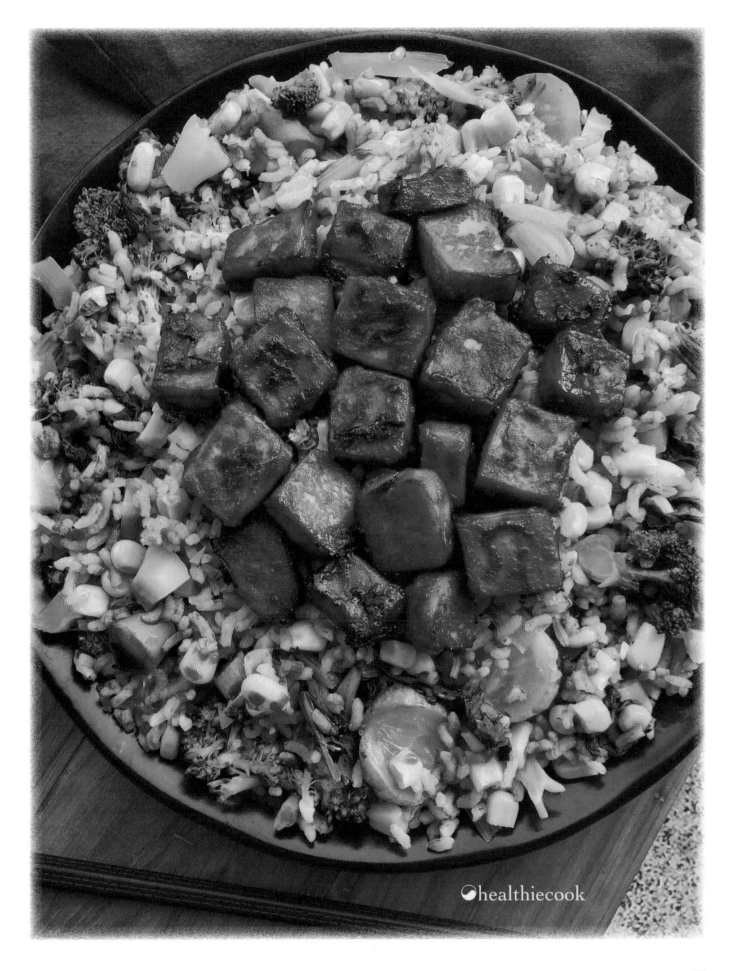

healthiecook

# POTATO & CHICKPEA CURRY

2 medium potatoes, peeled & chopped
1 (about 15oz / 400 grams) can of chickpeas, drained & rinsed
1 cup vegetables (I used broccoli & carrots), chopped
2 cloves garlic, finely chopped
1/2  medium onion, finely chopped
1 tbsp curry powder
1/2 tsp smoked paprika powder
black pepper & chilli powder, to taste
1 tbsp coconut sugar
1/4 cup coconut milk
1/4 cup tomato paste
water/vegetable stock, as needed
1 cup dry rice, cook according to package instructions, to serve

1. Bring a pot of water to a boil, add in the potatoes & carrots, boil until tender. Add in the vegetables, boil until cooked. Drain and set aside.
2. In a small bowl, mix together: coconut milk, tomato paste, curry powder, smoked paprika, coconut sugar.
3. Heat a non-stick pan (or add a bit of water to your pan to not use oil) over medium heat. Add in the garlic & onion, cook until fragrant.
4. Add in the curry mixture into the pan, mix in the cooked potatoes & vegetables, chickpeas until everything is fully combined. Add in some water/stock as needed to reach your desired thickness.
5. Enjoy with some freshly steamed rice, and there you have a delicious, nourishing, vegan meal!

**Credit:** *@healthiecook*

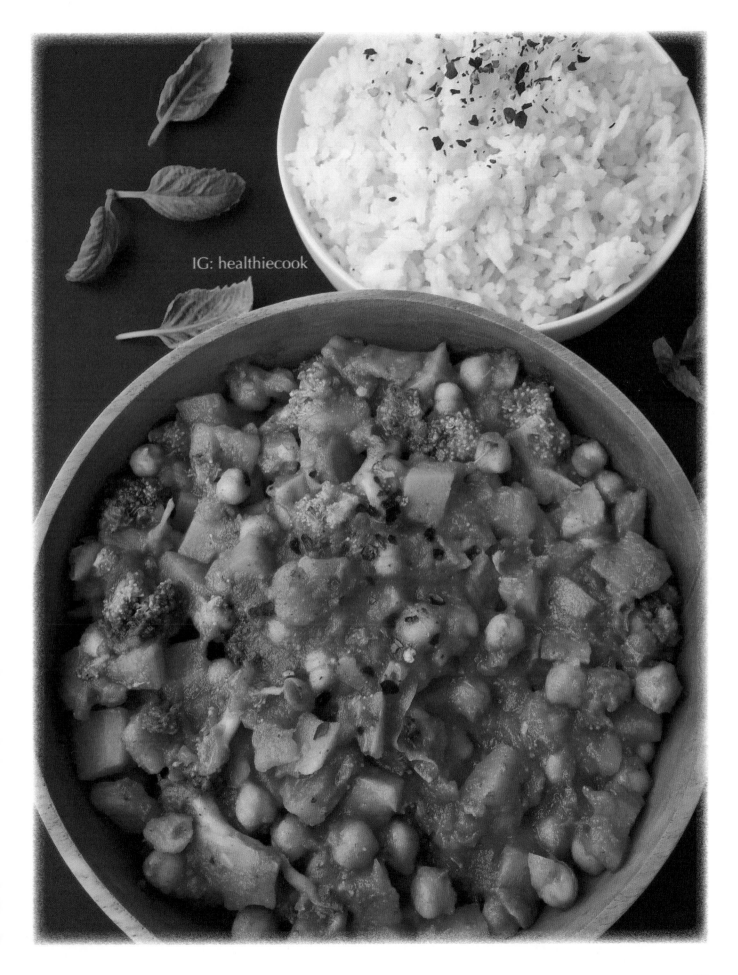

IG: healthiecook

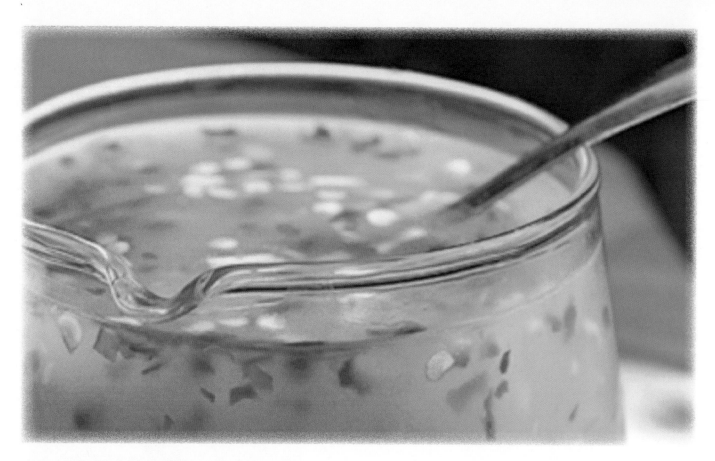

# SWEET CHILLI SAUCE

**1/2 cup Coconut Sugar**
**1/4 cup Water**
**3 Chilli's**
**1 Stalk Spring Onion**
**1/4 cup juice from Lime or Lemons**
**Optional: 1tbsp Potato Starch**

1. Finely chop the chilli and spring onion.
2. In a saucepan on a low to medium heat, add the chilli, coconut sugar and 1/4 cup of water.
3. Now stir the mixture frequently for about 3 mins to ensure no burning as this will give the sauce a bitter taste.
4. Add the spring onions and lemon/lime juice and cook for a further 5 mins.
5. Take it off the heat and let it cool for 10 mins or place it in the fridge until cool.
6. Optional, if you want a thicker consistency, you can add potato starch before you add in the spring onion.

**Credit:** *@freelee*

# LEBANESE PIZZA

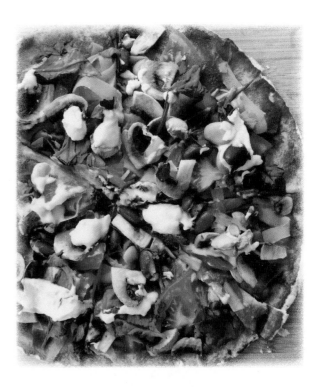

**2 Lebanese Bread**
**1 cup Pasta Sauce - Low Sodium / low fat**
**1 cup Mushrooms**
**2 tbsp Hummus (vegan)**
**1 cup Spinach**
**1 Tomato**

1. Preheat and oven or grill on medium heat.
2. Get the lebanese bread and spread the pasta sauce on it, then place the chopped mushrooms, spinach and tomato on top.
3. Cook until the bread is toasted and the vegetables are cooked.
4. Top with the hummus.

**Credit:** *@tianaaaxx*

# HOMEMADE TOMATO SAUCE

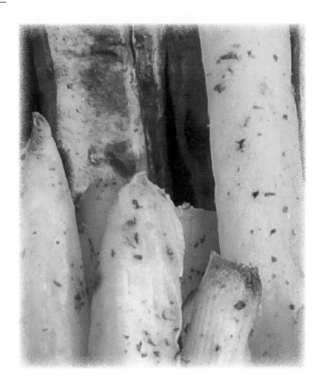

**2-3 tbsp 100% Tomato Paste (i.e. no added salt)**
**1 tsp Lemon Juice**
**1 tbsp Coconut Sugar**
**Optional: Chilli Flakes**

In a bowl, add in 2-3tbsp 100% tomato paste, 1tsp lemon juice, 1 tbsp coconut sugar and chilli flakes (optional).

*Note: Adjust all ingredients to taste – you may prefer it to be sweeter or more tangy

**Credit:** *@thrivingonplants*

# FINAL THOUGHTS

So, you can see that RT4 is not just a diet; it's a lifestyle. True health is a lifestyle. What I want for you is a healthy life in EVERY way, and that starts by taking care of yourself. It extends from there to your relationship with your partner, and your friends and family. It extends even further, to your relationship with the other species we share this planet with, and even further to your relationship with the planet itself. True health is living in balance inside and out. It means living in tune with nature. It means enjoying life. Finding happiness and true purpose in life, not because of some crazy idea that it comes from a certain body-type or from money or fame or other bullshit but finding TRUE happiness and purpose on your life journey from looking after yourself and others.

With these RT4 Principles you can begin to set yourself up with the foundation for a truly happy healthy life. Once you start on the journey and fully commit to it, you'll never stop growing and learning. You'll continue to improve on your health and your fitness with every step. I've been living this way for years, and I'm still improving every day. I'm not happy because of how I look; I'm happy because I'm in love with this journey. I'm in love with carbs. I'm in love with health and fitness, and I'm living a life of gratitude and purpose. Apply these principles to your life, cultivate an attitude of gratitude, try to live for something meaningful, and fall in love with the journey too! And I'll see you along the way :)

And remember... Be yourself and speak your mind because those who mind do not matter, and those who matter do not mind!

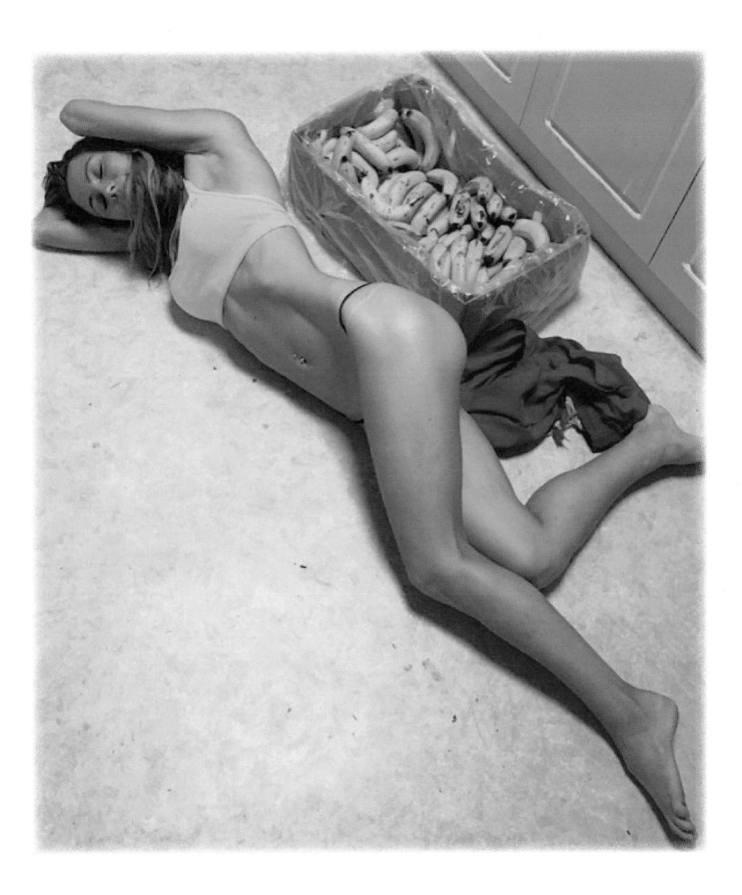

Printed in Great Britain
by Amazon

18736123R00123